WOLF SPIRIT

WOLF SPIRIT

A *Story of Healing, Wolves and Wonder*

By Gudrun Pflüger

Translation by Tammi Reichel,
APE International

RMB

RMB | Rocky Mountain Books Ltd.

rmbooks.com
@rmbooks
facebook.com/rmbooks

Cataloguing data available from Library and Archives Canada
ISBN 978-1-77160-127-6 (bound)
ISBN 978-1-77160-128-3 (epub)

Cover photos © Andreas Kreuzhuber (top) and Peter A. Dettling / terramagica.ca (bottom)
Printed and bound in Canada

Distributed in Canada by Heritage Group Distribution and in the U.S. by Publishers Group West

For information on purchasing bulk quantities of this book, or to obtain media excerpts or invite the author to speak at an event, please visit rmbooks.com and select the "Contact Us" tab.

RMB | Rocky Mountain Books is dedicated to the environment and committed to reducing the destruction of old-growth forests. Our books are produced with respect for the future and consideration for the past.

We acknowledge the financial support of the Government of Canada through the Canada Book Fund and the Canada Council for the Arts, and of the province of British Columbia through the British Columbia Arts Council and the Book Publishing Tax Credit.

Nous reconnaissons l'aide financière du gouvernement du Canada par l'entremise du Fonds du livre du Canada et le Conseil des arts du Canada, et de la province de la Colombie-Britannique par le Conseil des arts de la Colombie-Britannique et le Crédit d'impôt pour l'édition de livres.

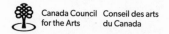
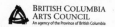

For NAHANNI,
My constant, "my girl,"
and all her wild relatives.

and

CONRAD KIMII,
My sunshine,
and all the children of his generation.

I love you.

Contents

Foreword

In Wildness is the preservation of the world.
—HENRY DAVID THOREAU, "WALKING"

What comes to mind when you hear the word "wolf?" Red Riding Hood and dark forests? Sharp teeth and danger? Unmodern creatures that no longer have a place in our contemporary society and landscape?

Or do you think of a gentle encounter that can save your life?

This is my story. There are as many stories as there are people. Many remain silent, some tell their stories, and a few set them down in writing. At the beginning I thought writing this story would be easy. Just describe one year after the other, nice and linear. But life isn't a straight line, and different experiences have such different significances and relationships to each other that a strictly chronological order didn't seem right. So I've chosen a structure that is more in keeping with the complex fabric of life and doesn't give the factor "time" any more importance than it actually has in my life. I don't even own a clock, and in the wilderness of Canada and during my illness, time played no role at all; there was only being or no-longer-being.

My motivation to write this book is my deep connection with everything natural and simple. Wolves are among those things. They are simply animals. But as soon as we start to use them as a surface on which to project our own fears and weaknesses, they become problematic animals that need to be driven away or even exterminated.

My experiences with wolves are not problematic. Thanks to them, I was able to perceive my love of life, strengthen my will to survive, and nourish my respect for all life.

Without my intense experiences in the wilderness, which often brought me to my very limits, I wouldn't have known how far my own strengths extend and where they actually come from. In untamed nature, I learned to respect that which is uncontrollable, to accept it, and finally recognize it as an essential part of my own life.

While I struggled with my illness, I coined the term "wolf spirit" to unite all the powerful qualities of wolves – their determination and endurance, their cohesiveness as a team, their joy, and their will to live. When I identified with the wolf spirit, I was successful in my own healing.

We urgently need to do everything in our power to preserve the natural habitats that still exist, not only for the sake of biodiversity but also for the well-being of our own souls. All our life force has its origins in unfettered nature. This message is, for me, inseparably connected with the wild, free-roaming wolves of Canada.

Prologue

FALL 1997

The city of Salzburg. Mozart is omnipresent. It's another of those rainy days in Salzburg. People who are familiar with the city will know what I'm talking about. Between two lectures at the university I stop by a nearby shopping centre where you can get good *topfenstrudel*, an Austrian cheese pastry. I still have a little time, so I let myself get drawn into conversation with a couple of people working for the animal protection organization *Vier Pfoten* (Four Paws). That's not usually my style, but sometimes things happen for a reason. These people work with attention-grabbers, shocking images of animals held in brutal conditions on fur farms or large-scale factory farms, pictures of skinned carcasses, caged four-legged circus artists, and animals that came to torturous deaths in traps. Images that are intended to engage people's emotions and spur them to action. What you think about those kinds of attention-grabbing techniques is secondary here. What's important is that there are people like that, who get involved in matters bigger than they are. I sign a membership card.

In one of their magazines I read a report about a wolf research and information project in the Canadian Rocky Mountains. I decide to sponsor one of the female wolves being tracked there. Sponsors receive regular updates about "their" wolves. Her name is Chinook, and she leads me onto the trail of the wild wolves.

New Dimensions

KOOTENAY

ON THE TRAIL OF THE WOLVES
WINTER 2000–2001

"Where did you come from?" There's no human settlement far and wide, but nonetheless there is suddenly a little dog trotting along next to me, looking at me with the intense gaze typical of a border collie. He tilts his head, and in his dark button eyes I read, "Let's go!"

"Go home, buddy! I can't take you with me. I'm travelling the entire length of the national park and won't be back this way again!" The little dog doesn't care a bit and scampers playfully ahead of me. I notice the tag on his collar. His name is Murphy, actually Jesus Murphy, and he can be returned to the telephone number noted below his name. "All right, fine, come with me. I don't know where I would take you around here anyway."

The only sign of human existence appeared right after I got out of the car: an open meadow with a snowed-in lodge at its far end. No vehicles, no voices, no human beings. My research colleague Danny had brought me to the southern boundary of the conservation area in our "burrito," an old and unreliable Ford the colour of a Mexican tortilla roll that belongs to Kootenay National Park. I intend to cover the length of the national park on my cross-country skis, heading north along East Kootenay Fire Road and turning to the west at the first bridge over the Kootenay River to meet the highway, where Danny is supposed to pick me up at the end of the day. That's the plan.

To the north and the east, Kootenay National Park borders on the more famous Banff National Park, and it expands the protected area from Alberta into British Columbia. It's also sometimes called, in a somewhat derogatory way, the "Highway National Park." This is because it owes its creation not to the environmental activism of a far-sighted nature lover, but to the fact that during construction of the first road running east–west through the Canadian Rockies, the province of British Columbia ran out of money and had to turn to the government in Ottawa for an infusion of cash. The government agreed under the condition that, in exchange, British Columbia relinquish control of the land eight kilometres left and right of the new road to the federal Crown to create a national park. No sooner said than done.

Today, Highway 93 bisects Kootenay National Park lengthwise. The highway is the shortest connection between the cold prairie with the booming metropolis of Calgary and the milder climate of the Columbia Valley with expansive Lake Windermere. Many residents of Calgary race quickly to their second homes on the lake or to the Panorama ski areas on the weekends, and few of them stop along the way. Most tourists limit their visits to Banff, and Jasper as well, and so Kootenay Park – aside from the terrible highway – remains relatively tranquil. The road is straight and is not fenced. The death toll among the wildlife is extremely high.

At the park's halfway point is Kootenay Crossing, where a park ranger lives, park road crews and the seasonal fire fighters are stationed (in summer), and there is a little bunkhouse that sometimes houses scientists working in the park. The nearest stores are in Radium Hot Springs in the Columbia Valley, 70 kilometres away. For a few weeks now I've been living in the bunkhouse, and I recently started sharing it with Danny and his old, broccoli-eating Labrador, Barkley.

Carolyn Callaghan, the leader of the Central Rockies Wolf Project, based in Canmore, about 120 kilometres away, has sent me into the Kootenay National Park. "Gudrun, our wolf Willow has disappeared. She was the only animal in the Kootenay pack with a radio collar. Now it's difficult to locate the rest of the wolves.

I expect that we'll have to cover a lot of ground looking for her. So I'd like to transfer you to Kootenay Park. You're good on skis and it doesn't bother you to work alone in the field." That was the beginning of an eventful winter and my training as a field researcher.

According to the map, the stretch I intend to cover today is 24 kilometres. I calculate: for that distance I need two hours, so with detours to look for tracks and breaks to enter data in the GPS system, maybe three. My experience has been that I cover 15 kilometres per hour, calculating generously. Or should I say according to European calculations, on well-groomed cross-country trails? Here, I sink into the snow with every step; there's no gliding at all. And after the first kilometre, I'm already questioning the function of the fire road, which is to ensure that firefighters have quick access to forest fires on the left bank of the river: trees stand close together, and I either crawl under them on my hands and knees or climb over them. The thick branches make everything even more difficult. Soon I'm sweating and cursing, especially after a glance at the GPS device tells me that after another hour I've only covered 1.4 kilometres. Every new time calculation pushes my arrival time dangerously late and I get nervous. I have no choice but to push forward. I have to make it to the bridge, today.

My worries don't seem to bother Murphy in the least as he bounds energetically ahead of me. But suddenly he stops as if he were frozen and fixates on the thick brush 2 metres ahead of us. His barking gets aggressive, which makes me uncertain. "What's got you so excited, Murph? Come on, let's go. We have to keep going. We still have a helluva long way to go." The little dog remains rooted to the spot. I start waving my poles in the air to loudly and firmly drive away this spirit behind the branches. After a few minutes, Murphy calms down and I can convince him to continue. Not 10 metres beyond the curve in the trail, we come across very fresh cougar tracks. So it was a cougar. I turn to Murphy and let out a deep sigh of relief. "Jesus, Murphy. You just did me an enormous favour." In the thickly snow-covered forest, I would never have known the animal was there. Like all cats, the cougar stalks its prey, mainly from behind and very quiet on its paws – in spite of its weight of up to a hundred kilograms. It is a master of secrecy. And I find it uncanny.

Two weeks later there is a tragic incident on a frequently used trail near Banff. A young woman goes cross-country skiing by herself and doesn't come back. Traces of blood and dragging are found, as well as the dead skier in the underbrush a few metres off the trail. And cougar tracks. Later the park rangers identify the likely killer; it's emaciated and sick and therefore displayed clearly abnormal behaviour. Nonetheless, it's a shock for all of us.

Thank heavens I don't know anything about this yet during my tour with Murphy, and anyway, I have other concerns: the light is slowly leaving us, and I still can't establish a radio connection with anyone. Even Murphy is showing the first signs of exhaustion. But we are on our own, and every step I don't take now will be missing at the end. I experience for the first time – as I will many times in the future – that time has only one dimension. Not past and future, not even present, but only "being" determines my entire concept of time.

Such extreme situations, experienced alone, push my boundaries. Every time I find myself in a tough situation, remembering other thorny moments from the past gives me renewed strength to make it this time too.

Once, while taking a shortcut, I broke through the ice on the Kootenay River, and immediately the strong current of the mountain river took hold of my entire body. I was in all the way. The ice water paralyzed me, but my thoughts were crystal clear: Get out fast, somehow! I grabbed the edge of the ice with both upper arms, hardly able to resist the force of the water. I knew that if I lost my grip, it would wash me under the cover of ice, which would surely mark my end. The ice edges held. Carefully, yet quickly, I pushed myself up onto them, hoping and praying. At first I pushed my chest slowly forward. The ice held. Lying flat with my arms and legs stretched out, I scooted toward the saving shore.

My guardian angel remained with me. After all, my car could

have been parked hours away, but it was actually within sight. When I reached the car, all of my clothing was frozen stiff. And again my angel didn't abandon me, because it only takes five minutes to drive to the place where I was staying. When I arrived there, she fluttered away and left me to a hot bath.

I soon trained myself not to take such shortcuts. Because there is always a very good reason for the normal route, for the path that local wildlife determine with their trails through the woods. They are familiar with the chasms and steep ledges, the swamps and the truly impenetrable places. Nothing in nature is random – everything has its logic and origins. Over time I, too, learn to recognize and understand these connections. And a new inner path comes about.

At some point on this particular journey with Murphy – and the exact time is totally unimportant – the outline of the eagerly anticipated bridge appears before me. I can radio to Danny, but he's already searching for me anyway. Murphy and I both sink into the seat of the car, quite exhausted. I will never again apply my old, familiar calculations of time and distance to the Canadian wilderness! I've learned that the hard way now. Danny just shakes his head. "I told you you'd never make it in three hours. We're in Canada!" He calls the ranger station to call off the alarm; they had already been alerted.

At home, Barkley gives up a couple scoops of dog food for Murphy and has to eat more broccoli for the next two days. That's how long it takes Jesus Murphy's owner to come and pick him up. When the car pulls up and Murphy's owner steps out, the little dog jumps up joyfully. Murphy's friend, Lyle Wilson, is good looking, in his mid-50s, dressed for the outdoors, with a youthful appearance and a dynamic presence. A George Clooney, only more attractive. I make a cup of coffee for him, the first of many, many hundreds we'll drink together in the coming years. And he begins to talk. We laugh a lot. It turns out to be a meeting with destiny. After just a few minutes, we realize that we could have met each other ten years earlier, in Finland, at the Nordic Junior World Ski

Championships. Lyle was there as coach of the Canadian women's team, I as an athlete for Austria. We're on the same wavelength; we notice it immediately. When he finally loads his dog into his car late in the day, he turns around one more time to say, "And get in touch! You know where we are now!"

During the winter in Kootenay National Park, I regularly drive to Carolyn in Canmore to take part in training for us field researchers, or just to do some shopping and be among people. Danny drives this stretch frequently too, to see his girlfriend. Sometimes we are visited by Mel, Melanie Percy, an experienced field biologist who gives us on-site tips. But even if the distances are vast here, I always have the feeling I'm in good hands, and I notice how tightly our common goals and interests bond us together.

All trackers work according to strict moral principles. We refer to following tracks as "back tracking," because as soon as we come across tracks, we follow them not toward the animal but in the opposite direction. Our motto is: the best research takes place when the objects of study never know they're being observed. Only then will they behave naturally, not influenced by us. For the information we need, it doesn't matter which direction we go, so we follow the wolves backward. You just have to think the other way around. When I find fresh, dark scat, for example, I know that I'll soon come across a kill; when I find a kill, I expect a hunting scene next. I save everything in the GPS device and upload it into the computer in the evening. Carolyn's main research focus is about when the animals overcome barriers. Such obstacles can be lots of things: rivers, fences, but especially roads. How does the wolf family behave when it reaches a road? That is, after all, the primary point of intersection between human activity and the everyday life of the wolves. And not a few of them, especially young, inexperienced animals, never reach the opposite side. We want to find out how regularly the pack crosses streets, where and how, in order to devise safe options for people and animals.

Whenever barriers pop up, the unity of the pack dissolves into a collection of individualists. Each animal overcomes the obstacle in his or her own way. A few stay calm and march right across it, some cross diagonally, and others turn around and run along the edge of the road for a few metres; others slip back into the forest and only reappear again when most of their comrades are already on the other side of the road and then they scurry to follow, employing a few quick bounds. The moments when I see the varied personalities of individual wolves written in the snow are especially fascinating to me.

On days following fresh snowfall, when the crystals at the surface of the snow sparkle under the winter sun like millions of the most precious diamonds, only interrupted by a trail of wolf paw prints like a string of pearls, I could look for hours at this beautiful painting that nature has placed before me. And then I often can't bring myself to ruin it with my own big boot prints. It's just too beautiful for me to plunge into. I'm overcome with so much respect for these animals and how their tracks fit into the landscape that I create my own path next to them. Humans don't always have to make the last brushstroke.

For a long stretch, the highway in Kootenay National Park follows the Kootenay River with its meanders, side arms, and sandbanks, with its steep, high walls of glacial rock and gently rolling low meadows. Like every river on Earth once was, and really always should be, it is a lifeline. Wild animals wander along its course, and plants carried by its current flourish. The dynamics of nature are evident. I love this river, especially because it's so varied and full of life, and so many messages are pressed into the sand of its banks. Whenever I get the chance to paddle down it – a few years later I even guided tourists on this river – I discover the park anew. Travelling along a waterway has always been the relatively easiest means through the wilderness. The human settlement of western North America followed the course of rivers. They were the primary travel routes for the First Nations and later "discoverers" as well. The Kootenay wolves also follow the river's course and take me to places in the park I would never have seen if it weren't for them. Even in my first winter in Kootenay National Park, I sensed that following wolves also means trustingly going in an unknown direction.

WOLF SPIRIT I
APRIL 2006

The morning sun shines through the train window, giving the fresh spring green of the Bavarian fields an additional, luscious layer of colour. Everything looks so clean and orderly, straight out of a kitschy tourism brochure. A few cows lie in the fields, basking in the first warm rays of sun, and some crows pick their breakfast out of those same pastures. The snow-covered Alps slowly but surely recede into the distance. The morning hours are especially beautiful at this time of year, when the great annual renewal is paired with the smaller, everyday awakening. The primroses and crocuses open their blossoms and greet the sun. The fruit trees are also full of blooms and transform themselves into terrestrial imitations of the white clouds in the clear, blue sky. Scattered farms blend into the gently rolling landscape, and the few larger towns along the way are practically swallowed by the lush nature.

The train stops and several young people get in; it is time for schoolchildren and working people to be under way. Two talkative young women settle into the seats diagonally opposite me. As one of them falls into her seat, she pulls her makeup kit out of her bag and begins to devote herself intently to her beautification. She and the rest of the train compartment, willing or not, are entertained by her friend, who tells us about the owner of a white Mercedes who wants to sue a young guy and his mother because he discovered a tiny black dot on his luxury car. Across from me sits a young man wearing an overdose of manly aftershave. Those who manage to ignore the chatter and the smell stare straight ahead, bored. Do they do this every day? Is this the way a large part of us humans begin the day in our society? While out there on the other side of the train window everything is eager for the new day and life? Am I the only one who finds everything around her exciting and so precious that I want to soak it all in, like a child? I am still perceptive, still interested in the environment. After all, I've just arrived from Canada, back to Central Europe, this land of excess. I've returned from a world that doesn't yet overwhelm our senses to the same degree, where it's still easy to perceive, to hear, to smell and feel what our sensing organs were created for, what they've adapted to over millennia, helping us survive in the process. And they are the reason that we can still feel like humans.

How wealthy are we really? And how impoverished? What have we achieved and what have we lost? What should we get used to and what should we never, ever be without? What should we accept and what should we rebel against? What does every human being need to be human?

Train thoughts. And the tracks bring me straight to my destination. It's that simple. Sit down in the right train and then arrive, without alternatives. If only life itself were so simple and straightforward.

I reach the destination of my train journey, the village of Markt Berolzheim in northern Bavaria, just south of Nuremberg. Everything is romantic here – it always surprises me that Germany can be so rural. Children play in the street, which is more like a country lane, and two little bakeries provide the inhabitants with the essentials. And then there's the big, old building directly next to the neighbouring in-town farmer's dung heap. Originally the parsonage, this building was beautifully renovated and now houses the practice of Dr. Arno Thaller. It is home to the hopes of many cancer patients from around the world.

In the Rhythm of the Tides

COASTAL RAINFOREST

MESSAGE IN THE AIR
SEPTEMBER 2001

Finally! Finally it's time. I'm on my way to the ancient red cedar. In the coming night, she will protect me from wind and rain with her long, dancing branches while I wait for wolves to fish at daybreak. In the last moments of daylight, I anchor the little boat in the isolated bay. I shoulder my backpack and carefully make my way toward the cedar. The rocky shore between the mouth of the river and the dense forest is very narrow right now. It's high tide and the ocean has reclaimed this piece of land that it will spit out again six hours later – embellished with lots of "goodies," nutrients from the ocean. Twice a day, the ocean bestows these gifts on this section of the coast, and when it has receded again, the animals of the forest and the air come to the richly set table in the intertidal zone.

Especially now, in mid-September, the ocean pushes millions of salmon ahead of it into the estuary, which waits for the fish like an open mouth. From the perspective of the salmon, however, the whole process has a few small flaws: they have to swim upriver, against the sometimes merciless current, even jumping up waterfalls using all their might. For us the Pacific salmon migration is always a breathtaking natural spectacle, but it's a deadly experience for the salmon. The terrestrial animal realm anticipates it each year with ravenous hunger: the bears have to eat enough to pack on their winter fat, the ravens are perpetually hungry, and the wolves also partake in this danger-free form of feeding by fishing at this time of year. The salmon that make it to their spawning grounds have just one advantage – albeit a decisive one – over those that become food for the predators a bit earlier: they may go to the eternal fishery knowing that they have reproduced. After they have spawned, they die.

The estuary where my cedar stands is smooth, because the terrain is flat. The river's current is gentle, and the water burbles calmly. But in between the gentle sounds I hear another noise, again and again at irregular intervals, that slowly swells and dissipates after a few seconds. It's the salmon, gathering their energy in small groups to swim another few metres against the current. Then it's quiet again for a short while before the fish finish their "breather" and proceed farther inland. At this time of day I hear and especially smell the fish in the river better than I can see them.

Unfortunately, the same is true of my cedar. The trees are just barely visible, and I only have a vague idea where it stands. My project leader, Chris, described it to me, but that was by daylight. Right. I do at least know that there's a rope hanging down from it, and that I have to use that to climb hand over hand to the first strong branch, and then upward along the thick side branches until I've reached the platform. The plan is good and logical; but in reality, it looks different. Darkness has engulfed the land. I feel my way and actually find a dangling rope, and because such infrastructure is relatively rare in a rainforest, I trust that I've gotten lucky, at least temporarily. And then I quickly realize I'll need a whole lot more good luck now. I am shouldering a sizable backpack with a sleeping bag and warm things. It has to go up the tree with me. As I climb, I can just dimly make out the next branch above my head, one at a time. At some point, the outline of a platform appears; after feeling around, I determine that it consists of nothing more than a few wooden boards nailed together – at least I hope so! – with generous spaces between them.

Since I promised myself on the climb upward that I most certainly wouldn't climb back down in the dark, my fate is sealed. With unconscious foresight, I brought along a rope that I now use to tie myself, in my sleeping bag, to the platform and the tree trunk, in the unlikely case that I nod off. And I do, very late at night. I wake in the early hours of the morning. The rhythmic sound of the slowly flowing river was the last thing I heard before drifting off, and it is now the first thing I hear. I concentrate and try to filter out any unusual noises. The sounds wolves make as they fish.

Slowly the first light settles onto the estuary. Now my work can begin: have wolves stationed themselves at the river to fish for salmon, as Chris observed at many previous dawns? I know the chances aren't very good; the tides are high. But you have to take the opportunities you're given. Now it starts to drizzle lightly. It's wet and cold. A hot sip from my Thermos feels good. Tentatively, the first outlines of the forest and the river meadow emerge from the receding darkness. It is that glorious hour when everything appears in different shades of blue. Mist rises silently from the river. Individual ravens and crows announce themselves. And suddenly they begin in the distance: slowly rising, then more and more, louder and louder. In a short time, the entire river valley is filled with the howling of wolves, drawn out, long and never-ending. I time it, then give up, because the howling just doesn't want to end. When it briefly breaks off, it begins again immediately. I've never experienced this kind of howling and am captivated by the wolf frequencies. There is something different about them, drawn out, plaintive – yes, it's plaintive. And the sound just doesn't end, or even come closer. It hangs in the trees, hovers above the river and thickens all the air in the valley. The birds are silent. It seems as though the whole world is holding its breath to listen to the message in the air.

Since the source of the howling isn't coming closer and the sky is slowly getting brighter, I have little hope of observing wolves this morning. I decide to leave my night camp and move to firm ground. I look down in disbelief. Where does this tree end? All I can see are branches and more branches, covered with thick layers of lichen and juicy green mosses – no ground to be seen anywhere. I start to climb down and have to swallow hard. I'm glad that I didn't see last night how far the fall through the gaps in the platform would have been.

The wolves' howling has ceased now and no longer fills the valley, but it echoes inside me in a strange way. I've heard a lot of howling before, but this chorus had an extra dimension. Deeply moved, I arrive at the little wooden dock of the McAllisters, my host family. Rob, a friend, is standing at the end of the dock and seems confused. That happens to Rob quite often. I want to tell him about my wonderful howling wolves experience right away, but when he starts to speak, I quickly realize he has unimaginable news: an airplane has flown right into the World Trade Center, everything exploded, total chaos in New York, another plane in Washington also exploded, all radio programs are interrupted and new bits of information are coming thick and fast.

I run up into the house, where everyone is sitting or standing around the radio, speechless, listening intently to the live reports from New York. In the next hours and days, all of us, just like the rest of the Western world, will painfully realize the incredible extent of the events of that morning (Pacific Standard Time) of September 11, 2001. I am dumbfounded, pull out my notes – yes, there's no doubt about it. The eerie howling of the wolves took place in the exact same moments in which a building, a world power and a worldview collapsed. What did the wolves out there in the secluded, peaceful river valley know and sense? That will always remain their secret. I, on the other hand, struggle to make sense of these two, so contrasting, simultaneous events.

In situations like this, it's impossible to believe in coincidences; it just doesn't work, there is too much unconscious knowledge and feeling involved. How can it be that at the exact same time when I felt so comfortable and securely bound up in nature, people were being attacked with human technology with such precision and efficiency? That at the same time I was filled with inner satisfaction and peace, so much hate and terror was brought into our world?

I have to think of the old wolf myths. After all, in many cultures, the wolf is honoured as an intermediary with the realm of the dead. People believe that wolves can travel back and forth between the worlds. And in the Old Norse *Edda*, the wolf symbolizes the end of the world or the defeat of the gods.

At the end of lectures about my work researching wolves, I am always asked if it isn't very dangerous to roam around alone in wolf and bear territory. Sometimes I answer this question with a short story about a rickety platform high up in an old cedar and the message in the air.

WASTEFULNESS
SUMMER 2002

"We'll just buy the regular milk and then we can add water to make it low fat. That'll save us some." Yoey rolls her eyes and I think to myself, "Chris, now you're going too far!"

We're standing in the famous/infamous Band Store in Waglisla, or Bella Bella, as the town is named on Canadian maps. Famous because it's the only grocery store on the island, and infamous because it's the only grocery store on the island: everything is expensive, and the produce suffers visibly from the long journey to get here. To save money, we stuffed Chris's small Toyota full of food back in Victoria. Every cubic centimetre that isn't occupied by our bodies, the many tools used for collecting wolf scat, toilet paper for ourselves – you can compare prices of some interesting things – or rain gear, is crammed with noodles, canned goods, heads of cabbage, or trail mix. Along the highway that runs through Vancouver Island we buy fresh fruit and vegetables, and on top of everything we balance a jar of honey straight from a beekeeper.

At the terminal for the ferries in Port Hardy, we have to reload everything on the Inside Passage ferry, which after a seven-hour trip spits us out again in McLoughlin Bay, the dock 2 kilometres from Waglisla. It's one in the morning. In the darkness, we once again unpack everything, bring the boxes to the little jetty where Ian is already waiting with his boat, load everything on the boat, and zoom across the dark sea to neighbouring Denny Island. There we unload the boxes one last time and carry them up to the small, but not particularly fine (although perhaps it once was, decades ago), green and white-striped cabin, referred to henceforth as the "sugar shack." The dock is an adventure in itself and has more holes than boards. It's also low tide, and the short climb to the cabin is very steep. But at some point the provisions are stashed in the pantry, toilet paper and all, and we lie down on our bunks of milk crates and boards.

During the next few days we do our best to spruce up our sugar shack and make it fit for human habitation. Later, two volunteers, Phil and Claire, also join our team. The cabin is full to bursting, but the atmosphere is fantastic. Claire decorates the walls with paintings; Yoey is our disc jockey and somehow always obtains what we need to keep the cabin in one piece. Phil cobbles together a rain-water-collection system out of a plastic tarp and a tub; he is our rainforest version of a freshwater collector. Once a week we can run a bath. After sniffing each other, we determine who bathes in what order: the cleaner ones first, then the ones that don't smell so good. No matter how much wood we put in the old iron stove, our sugar shack is and remains damp. At some point, Chris invests in our health and orders a big dehumidifier. Its container is full every day. I paint a big skull and crossbones on a poster and hang it on the door of our ancient refrigerator: if you touch it in the wrong place, it gives off electrical shocks that would knock out any bear on the island.

Yoey is a genuine coastal girl; she is always finding something useful floating on the water or on the beach. Beachcombing is an official job description for many on the West Coast: people slowly traverse the beaches, "combing" them in search of washed-up stuff. There's a lot of it. The true art of it is to imagine a purpose for a piece of torn-off rope or interestingly shaped boat parts. Like many others, Rob is especially on the lookout for good logs; people can recognize the quality of the wood by how deep they bob in the water, and it can be very good. But most of what piles up along the coast is useless, broken stuff, and just plain garbage. The Pacific is vast, and lots of people, entire cities and industrial complexes, dispose of their garbage in the ocean, supposedly never to be seen again.

In recent times we've learned that far away from all human eyes, a carpet of plastic covering more than a million square kilometres is floating in the middle of the Pacific. The plastic is slowly decomposing, and the particles hover in the ocean water like natural plankton. In the Pacific there are already six particles of plastic for every plankton. Fish and marine birds are thus "feeding" on more and more plastic. And eventually, if they don't die of the consequences before that, they land on our plates. Yes, the world is round, and the Canadian saying "what goes around, comes around" is also fitting. In earlier times, beautiful glass balls that Japanese fishers used as buoys, loosed from their fishing nets, would wash up on the western coast of Canada after a long journey by sea; today "presents" of another kind land here.

Ever since the nuclear reactor catastrophe at Fukushima in Japan, I think especially often of my friends on the coast and all the wild animals that feed themselves from the ocean and breathe the air of the westerly winds. If glass buoys from Japan once made it to the West Coast of North America …

Our garbage, i.e., everything we have produced and no longer need, is growing out of control. Unnecessary packaging is a symptom of our wasteful lifestyle. What we leave behind only creates problems. What is left over in nature, on the other hand, is an important component of the cycle of growth and decay. It isn't wasteful, for example, when the coastal wolves eat almost exclusively the heads of salmon and leave the rest lying on the shore. Numerous birds, small animals, and insects feed on the remains, and these carcasses that provide protein – and thus nitrogen – are essential to the plant life of the rainforest.

Or the remains of a wolf kill in the Rocky Mountains: I have to get very lucky to discover a kill quickly enough that all the other animals that benefit from the remains have left something behind. We've counted 28 other species of animals that serve as "clean-up crew," feeding on the carcass after wolves or even while wolves feast. Small rodents get valuable calcium from the bones, while the sassy ravens even try to grab the best pieces from the wolves.

There are also many tiny organisms, decomposers, which transform what's left over into smaller pieces, molecules or substance groups that can be used again. Again and again, I'm fascinated by the quick transformation of captured prey into new life. Nothing is wasted; nothing is left over; the whole cycle can start over again.

The Heiltsuk people were also self-sufficient or engaged in simple trade with tribes on the mainland until the arrival of Europeans. Later, the people used valuable glass beads as one would money. But the culture of the West Coast First Nations is fundamentally shaped by one resource above all: the western red cedar. They made their houses and boats from these trees, and clothing, blankets, storage containers, or rope from the bark and roots. And they peeled the bark so adroitly that the trees were never seriously damaged by it. Many of the once-harvested trees are still standing in the forests, and square or triangular indentations in their bark reveal their former usage. They remain silent witnesses of a respectful and responsible relationship between people and their resources.

Seaweed – an edible and very healthy kind of algae – herring roe, a few seagull eggs once in a while as a treat, mussels, and especially the valuable eulachon oil of the small, extremely fatty candlefish, but also the roots of several wild plants: everything was utilized with respect and awareness of its great value, and consumption was celebrated.

The Ktunaxa (Kootenay) First Nation west of the Rocky Mountains snuck over the high peaks every year into the territory of the Niitsitapi (Blackfoot) to hunt a few bison. They hauled every bone back over the steep paths into what is now the Columbia Valley. Everything was too precious to waste. It's estimated that every year in Germany between €10- and €20-billion worth of food, or as much as €235 per person, is thrown away. With the food that lands in the garbage in Europe, we could feed all the people in the world who go hungry – twice.[1]

Even during my first stay in this area, I noticed immediately

1 See *Taste the Waste*, directed by Valentin Thurn (Germany, 2011), DVD.

that people don't just happen to live on the Central West Coast. The few white people who have settled here live here for a reason, simply and in harmony with nature and the tides. Again and again I meet new characters, and each time they show me a new way to live. And somehow they all manage. Their motto, "What I don't need, I don't need to earn in the first place," allows a different pace of life. And when the storm tears away a dock somewhere, everyone shows up to build a new one together. Every individual is valuable, even the old guy who used to be the custodian at the fish cannery. He is the last inhabitant of the Brookdale settlement after the factory was closed. With his little boat and his two old huskies, Cash and Credit, he regularly docks at Shearwater Marina, two coves away from our sugar shack, to pick up his beer and hear the latest news. If there isn't any, there'll be some speculation about the new waitress at the only pub within a radius of a hundred kilometres. And that's usually the case.

Yoey's acquaintance Danny can do everything, and best of all are his jam sessions à la the Grateful Dead. Jerry, Mike, Louise, Lise – the list of Central Coast residents is not all that long. But their stories are colourful. It's a small world unto itself, where you don't need very much to be happy.

At the same time, though, Shearwater is the gateway to a contrasting world. With one of the few marinas along the Central Cost, it is a meeting point for the super-rich and their swimming luxury boats. We call them "Tupperware boats" because most of them are testaments to a lot of money and not much taste. Their owners disembark and buy a few things in the little grocery story. While they do their laundry, they make a trip to the pub or buy parts for their boats in the marine shop and have them replaced in the workshop. I actually like the crazy mix of such diverse types of people in such a small place. The surrounding sea gives you the feeling that there is enough room for everyone. For the frugal and the squanderers, the social critics and observers, the dropouts and the newcomers, those who embrace life and those who are taking a breather.

And the Shearwater Pub's halibut burger is a classic that we treat ourselves to after overnight trips, most of which are wet and cold. Our "boss," Chris, sometimes steps out of his normal role and treats the team to a round of burgers and beers at the pub. That turns a burger into something very special.

Ian and Karen McAllister, founders of the forceful and effective environmental organization Raincoast Conservation Foundation, have been living on Denny Island for ten years. Their operations are financed through supporters that include very wealthy foundations. Ian and Karen make it a point to cultivate a personal relationship with their financial backers. They are invited to take trips into the rainforest and stay overnight at the McAllisters' home. Over time, more and more supporters and international film crews show up. And parties are held, frequently, that begin with tables richly laid with salmon and other seafood, wine and even fresh fruit and vegetables, and end with energetic dancing in the living room. It is always such an intoxicating feeling to spend a few hours with like-minded people. We celebrate the cohesiveness and the contribution each of us makes, whether it's through scientific research or environmental protection efforts, reporting for the media or providing generous financial support. We are all on the same team. We shake hands all around, and each time, someone says thank you for the bounty of nature that's being shared with good friends.

At some point, nature calls and everyone has to find the facilities. At the McAllisters' there's a sign hanging above the toilet with a little reminder: "If it's yellow – leave it mellow. If it's brown – flush it down!" Even here, awareness is being raised, in this case about saving the resource of water. And that applies equally to everyone.

"Since we're out here anyway, let's just gather everything that seems interesting and important to us." Chris is far-sighted, engaged, and a true biologist. Everything is connected to everything else, and therefore any observation can potentially provide further information about why wolves do what they do. Fieldwork is extremely time-consuming, especially in this region. We quickly learn to make the most of our resources. Chris's alarm goes off at 6:00 am – for the first time. Because he still needs to snooze a little while longer. I, on the other hand, am immediately wide awake and curse his stupid routine, as I do every day. Eventually, Claire's and Phil's beds rustle too, and soon all of us schlep ourselves into the 10-square-metre kitchen–living room–dining room. Chris is the last one in. Yoey has installed herself in the "birdhouse" next to the sugar shack and comes over for breakfast.

While the coffee is brewing and the weather report runs, we talk about the work to be done that day. The teams are established. Since I am the only one besides Chris who knows the wolf trails, I tell Yoey something about them. Claire and Phil get some information about deer beds and hair. Chris goes with Lone Wolf, whose actual name is Chester Starr. We pick him up at the dock in Bella Bella. Chester is a member of the Heiltsuk Nation and supplies us with local knowledge about the weather, land and people. His relationship with time sometimes drives Chris up a wall: when Chester doesn't show up, it's probably because he drank too much the previous night. Then we pilot our *Mandarine*, our Double Eagle boat painted in that lovely colour, especially carefully. The water hides many rocks and reefs. Chester knows them all – even in fog, he always knows exactly where we are at any given moment. He still observes his environment very precisely. Like many Indigenous people, he still has this intimate relationship with nature and the landscape. There are some trips we only make when he is with us in the boat.

Once we've made land, we separate. Sometimes we are even on different islands, which almost led to a catastrophe once when Chris, who was alone and had the boat, was seriously pursued by a black bear and only escaped an attack by a hair's breadth by jumping into the boat. Yoey and I were on another island without a boat, and Phil and Claire were out of reach of radio reception. After that, no one went out alone for a long time. Even though in terms of efficiency, it is always very tempting to go searching for tracks on your own.

The great thing about being solo is that you move through the forest completely differently, much more attuned and attentive. And I always come back to the hut in the evening so full of impressions. I notice that Chris feels the same way, and even in our second season in the field, sometimes the two of us get nostalgic remembering the intensive days of the previous year. More than once we had crawled back to the little hut on the hill behind the McAllisters' house, where we both still lived at the time, and used our last bit of strength to tear open that North American affront to every bastion of gourmet food, and in two minutes made ourselves a Kraft macaroni dinner with unnaturally orange powdered cheese sauce. It was bad. Not even the pieces of broccoli tossed in to increase the vitamin content by 200 per cent could salvage that meal. Wet and chilled to the bone, we sank into the couch, knowing for sure we're victims of science.

But such experiences create bonds, and we are still the best of friends today, thanks to the structure of our human brains, which prefers to hang on to the nicer aspects of life and deposits the dubious experiences farther to the back. But they are still there and retrievable.

I remember the many depressing days, too. When I was out there alone, frozen and unsuccessful, and in the evenings, one question blocked any other thoughts: "Why exactly am I doing this, again?" A déjà vu moment from my years as an elite athlete. The tumour I was diagnosed with four years later provided the answer. Then, at the latest, the days become meaningful, not only the days when I was able to gather important data about wolves and their ecosystem, but especially the days when I didn't reach my goals, the days that I saw as wasted time at first: I needed them to catch my breath, to be able to look forward to a new day and concentrate on the next task. They are an important part of learning not to expect to find success behind the next tree. And to appreciate it when it does come. No, not one day was a waste of time.

WOLF SPIRIT 2
JULY 2005

Sunshine Meadows are in their full glory, full of flowers, and a grizzly bear grazes in the distance. It's a wonderful summer day.

Together with Magi and Sabrina, "Speedy Sab," I run over a pass from Sunshine into Brewster Valley and then out into the Bow Valley. I am delighted by this day, the beautiful blue sky, and my two friends, who are showing me a gorgeous part of Banff National Park that's new to me. The narrow hiking trail is uneven, with lots of protruding roots. That's never been a problem; on the contrary, I love challenging trails. Nonetheless, my right foot gets caught on small obstacles and I stumble repeatedly. Hardly noticeable at the time. When we take a break at a junction and have a drink, I want to say something but can't. I just can't get the words out. I know exactly what I want to say, have the sentence in my head, but I can't make the motions to speak it out loud. It irritates me a little, but I'm probably just dehydrated. I drink a lot, and we continue running. I avoid saying anything. The stumbling and stammering are embarrassing to me. That's it. Content with our accomplishment, and of course somewhat tired, we arrive at the parking lot.

A few weeks later, I'm running with a group of fit young men, friends of Phil, my boyfriend at the time. Afterward we all get a drink together, and I notice that my tongue and lower jaw don't want to obey me again. I can't get a word out. Again I drink a lot – I should get more fluids in general, races through my head. Meanwhile, Phil has been complaining for quite a while that I'm unfocused and clumsy. Things often fall out of my hands, or I spill drinks. I'm under some pressure due to my current job as a production assistant for the ZDF television film about my work with wolves on the West Coast, because I have to call complete strangers and ask them for support of all kinds. I'm learning a lot, but especially that I'm not good at making phone calls.

In spite of this inner pressure, I'm extremely excited about the late summer of 2005, when these efforts will finally pay off and I can return to the coast. Since spring I've been living with Phil in his apartment in Canmore. We got to know each other better during a crazy drive to a cross-country skiing race in Nipika. The roads were blocked due to ice, and the long detour gave us plenty of time. Although he is deeply involved in cross-country skiing – while I want to leave my past behind me – and even coaches a company team, I like him a lot. He is both a very reliable and a crazy-fun partner. He is smart and likes to design and tinker with things. A typical raven, I think, when we both visit a shaman who helps us get acquainted with our totem animals. Phil would never have gone for that kind of "voodoo," as he calls it, on his own; I practically had to drag him. But we all – even my sister Gerhild, who was with us – took a lot away from it.

My work on the film project with ZDF lets all other frustrations fall to the wayside, and finally the day comes when I can pack my things and fly to the coast. For the first two weeks, I am supposed to scout for filming locations with Jean Marc on his sailboat, the *Tilsup*, before the filming crew arrives. Those turn out to be the best two weeks of all my time in the rainforest. Early on, Jean Marc brings me to an island off the coast that has a wonderful, wide, white sand beach. I am so full of life and energy, so content and fulfilled. On the boat I laugh a lot with and at Jean Marc, and together we comb the beaches of the isolated island looking for flotsam and make a game out of suggesting what it might still be used for.

Then the US-American wildlife cameraman Jeff and his assistant Karin (now his wife) join us; they add even more to our high spirits. We are on the same wavelength, make excursions to beaches together and discuss everything under the sun. We sail along shores and bays. I hop off the boat, look for fresh wolf tracks, jump back on board, and do the same thing again in the next bay. Even as a child I would get slightly carsick, and now I live on swaying boats. I am constantly slightly nauseous, and on land I stumble more and more often over the big, slippery rocks on the shore. Of course, I ascribe my increasing clumsiness to the constant change between land and boat, lack of sleep, and the strenuous days of filming. No other explanation occurs to me.

HIGH SEAS
SUMMER 2001

"Are you sure your boat can't flip over?" I scream up to Jean Marc somewhat hysterically. We call him JM, the best skipper on the seven seas. The storm whips my words into his ears, and he bends down a little from the helm into the galley, where I try to hold tight as if I were a gecko with suction cups and try not to fly through the small room along with the dishes, books and food. The *Tilsup* is leaning, and has been for much too long for my landlubber legs. JM's wonder-sailboat made of aluminum is sunk to the railing in the wild, black sea.

"Nearly sure," he yells at me.

"Nearly is not enough right now!" I scream back, and withdraw to the farthest corner of the boat.

Erin comes from the prairies, far from the stormy ocean. Together we curse in our sleeping-berths. Erin pulls up the safety net on the side of her bunk right away. I look at her with concern and consider whether I should do that too – Bam! – and land like a piece of wood on the floor of the ship. Okay, I can't get any lower. I just won't move again until the storm is over or we end up in the eternal fishing ground. Twyla, the energetic filmmaker on board, is also a passionate diver. She lives in and on the ocean; it's her element. Currently she is making her way along the boom on the open deck, ·hand over hand, toward the stovepipe, which the storm has just lifted off its foundation. Hopefully she isn't the next to go! I am paralyzed with fear, and horrific scenarios race through my mind. Ever since I almost drowned in a swimming pool as a three-year-old – and I can still remember the minutes spent underwater very clearly – I've had a troubled relationship to everything associated with water. And now I'm leading the team carrying out a large-scale study of wolves along the islands off the coast of British Columbia. Ten days ago we set out from Bella Bella with two sailboats to search an area of more than 20,000 square kilometres for signs of wolves. Chris and his crew are sailing with the second boat, the *Nawaluk*, between the mainland and the coastal islands, while we – for better or worse – are cruising along between the western coast of the coastal islands and Japan, and, for a time, Haida Gwaii, the Galápagos Islands of the North.

At the start of the expedition, I know nothing of the wild storms, jagged rocky beaches and the great difficulty of even landing on the islands. As soon as I stretch so much as my little toe outside, I am already soaking wet. Nonetheless, or maybe because of this – it's a well-known fact that people come together in a crisis – we are always in top spirits, not least because of JM, the greatest character along the entire Pacific Coast. Sometimes he turns around to face us and we stare into a blood-red eye; sometimes he replaces his lower arm with a hook, then suddenly pulls frighteningly realistic beasts and giant clam muscles out of the stovepipe, or even worse, out of the cooking pot. His supply of pirate accessories seems to be endless. Of course, he also keeps harmless things like pirate flags with skull and crossbones and a treasure chest, just to complete the collection.

JM worked on his *Tilsup* for almost three years before he was ready to let her down from the stocks. She is the most unique sailboat under the sun. Wherever we moor, heads turn to look: her aluminum-silver and the giant squid painted on her deck, the pirate flag waving overhead, and psychedelic music coming from the loudspeakers are anything but typical. What really impresses everyone, though, is how JM can park his boat with millimetre precision between two docked boats. Two independent motors make the *Tilsup* as agile as a cat. Together with her skipper, she amazes the boating world. No other skipper could ever have brought us to the places that are possible with JM. He loves challenges, surprises, diving, his bachelor lifestyle, his guitar, vegan food and going barefoot. Because he has turned his back on an uncritical consumer society, he is forward thinking and extremely open to the world. Everyone knows JM, and everyone loves him. JM is simply JM.

Before the start we agreed to meet the *Nawaluk* at the halfway point in Bernard Harbour. There are nine of us on board the *Tilsup*: JM, "southern Chris" (director of the Raincoast Conservation Foundation), Twyla and her boyfriend/filming assistant Jeremy, Anne (a volunteer helper), Erin, Lone Wolf, Marven of the Gitga'at First Nation, and me.

Erin has come to the coast for about a month, purely due to her interest in research techniques. She wants to start a master's degree program next year and gather her genetic data set from wolf scat. After just a short time, we are already calling each other "sister." When she begins her research in Prince Albert National Park in the winter of 2003, I become her supervising field biologist.

But for now, I am extremely excited about this meeting with the *Nawaluk*. We are not entering Bernard Harbour bay unprepared. JM's pirate chest is filled with our treasures: wolf scat and even a wolf's skull from a skeleton we found curled up peacefully underneath a huge cedar. In the past few days, Erin and I also put our musical talents to the test, rewriting a song by Ben Harper and teaching it to the rest of the crew. JM and Twyla accompany us on their guitars. Before we tie the *Tilsup* to the *Nawaluk*, our group assembles on the deck and puts on a show. At the end of the song comes Lone Wolf's solo performance: a long, drawn-out howl. Then we hand over our treasure chest to the crew of the *Nawaluk*.

We spend the rest of the day sitting together on the larger *Nawaluk*, talking about what we've experienced. Not that I expected anything different: Chris and his group have hardly had any bad weather, certainly no storms, but instead have video cameras full of footage of wolves at several rendezvous points. Greedy and a little envious, I watch their films. We have seen wolves one single time, two of them. I don't hold it against the wolves, of course; in such an inhospitable place, I would also withdraw to the side of the island with friendlier weather as fast as possible. Once, Paul even says, "We anchored right in front of their rendezvous and the wolves were on the beach the whole time. At some point, it got kind of boring to watch them." I'd love to have that problem sometime.

I met Paul, Dr. Paul Paquet, for the first time in the basement of Carolyn Callaghan's house in Canmore, which was also the office of the Central Rockies Wolf Project. His warm, patient and highly competent energy immediately fascinated me. He gives the most inexperienced students the same respect and attention as a world-famous scientist. His big heart has enough room for everyone who works to protect the environment and wildlife, or for the preservation of Native cultures and traditional knowledge. He has established a reputation worldwide as a large-carnivore conservationist, is associate professor at several universities, and sits on the council or board of directors for many organizations, including WWF Worldwide. Nonetheless, when you stand before him, his world revolves entirely around you. In any case, this encounter in the basement was a life-changing, fateful moment: I was a volunteer tracking Kootenay wolves, and the winter was slowly coming to an end. The first snow-free patches heralded the end of the season for following tracks in the snow, and my inner voice repeated over and over again: *Gudrun, you're at home here. This gives your life meaning and satisfaction. You feel strong here. Stick with it!* And then Paul stood before me for the first time, the man who has a hand in every significant project having to do with large predatory animals. From that point on, all of my work has taken place under his aegis. In the coming years, he and his wife Anita become something like my adoptive parents. I celebrate Christmas and New Year's with them and their international, intellectual artist friends in sweet little Meacham, a prairie village in Saskatchewan. One time, I happened to be with them when Paul heard the news that his good friend Erik Zimen, Germany's most famous wolf researcher, had collapsed suddenly while giving a lecture. A short time later, we knew why: a brain tumour. Erik died less than two months later. A few years earlier I had visited Erik at his farm in the Bavarian Forest, renovated in a homey Swedish style. After that he wrote me a very encouraging letter. I learn of his death from Paul, on the phone. Paul is beside himself, and for some strange reason the news affects me very deeply. Like a kind of foreshadowing. And three years later, when I have to call Paul, all he says is, "Not again," and starts to cry.

The next day, our boats go their separate ways. Our day together was my birthday, and we celebrated late into the night. Anita managed to conjure up a birthday cake, and in the middle of nowhere, Paul presented me with a bouquet of beautiful (fresh) flowers!

There were even a few little presents for me to unwrap. Erin gathered a few berries every time we went on land and made a jar of jam out of them. And so it was that thanks to my incredible friends, I celebrated my most wonderful birthday party to date on a boat in the wilderness of Canada.

The *Tilsup* sets course to the northwest, where there are two small islands 12 kilometres from any other land mass. We are curious but don't expect very much: how should wolves be able to live on these islands, and above all, how would they have reached them in the first place? The islands have the characteristics typical of the coastal islands: there are hardly any hills, they're overgrown with moss and small bushes, are home to many marshes, and just a few dwarfed, wind-whipped cedar trees give the horizon a structure. It is the second stage of the expedition, our volunteer's time has run out, and the crew has shrunk. The weather is stormy – how could it be any different? – so only Chester and I go ashore. After a short time, I can't believe my eyes: wolf scat. Is this really true? Can this be here? All other alternatives are excluded. I bend over the mound. In this solitary moment in a heavy downpour, I can't begin to imagine that these will become probably the most often-mentioned wolf droppings in the world. And yet this find proves for the first time that coastal wolves can swim up to 12 kilometres in the wild, cold Pacific, a masterful achievement that proves one thing above all: these wolves are extremely well-adapted to their environment. Here, where the sea is so closely intertwined with the land, both elements are a part of their habitat. And it is important to take good care of the sea and the land, and keep both of them healthy. Another question naturally arises as well: what other secrets do these wolves harbour that make them so special and make them and their habitat so important and worthy of protection? We are in year one of the Rainforest Wolf Project, and with every discovery, new questions come up.

In 2015 the project enters its 15th season. Teams and lines of questioning have changed over the years, but not the major recognition of the genetic and morphological uniqueness of these wolves and the main goal associated with that: to sustain this last intact section of coastal rainforest in the world, its inhabitants, and all the ecologically significant interactions taking place there. With each new discovery, the protection of such ecosystems becomes more significant, and the argument for their protection better grounded.

But the most important qualities of such regions probably aren't mentioned in any scientific reports. The ones that give us strength – giving meaning and joy to our lives – to continue to live for something, work for it – even fight for it. Those qualities that unite people who share the same values and literally allow them to cross the often turbulent seas together in one boat, to new shores.

TRADITIONS
WINTER 2002

Now the young wolf is prepared. For two years he learned from his parents and elder siblings. What they know, in turn, consists of knowledge handed down by their parents, supplemented by their own experiences. The same is true for his grandparents and their ancestors. In this way, the pool of knowledge becomes ever larger, more complex and more relevant.

The young wolf was born in an undisturbed den somewhere under one of the big, old cedars. He has no experience of human beings; his parents have never had to teach him about that subject. He does know exactly where to find the best salmon and the easiest ways to fish them out of the water. He can swim well and already has the rhythm of the tides in his blood. His knowledge is the accumulation of the experiences of his ancestors over millennia. Many of them grew old enough to pass down rich stores of information. His brethren of similar age in the comparatively densely populated regions of the southern Rocky Mountains in Canada are not in the same situation. For about two hundred years, experienced older wolves in that area have repeatedly been killed by humans. The pups are still in the middle of training when they lose their teachers. So they have to try to make their way the best they can on their own. Their hunting strategies aren't very well developed yet, and they often haven't quite figured out the principles that guide the behaviour of their prey, and what roads are all about remains a mystery. So they wander aimlessly on the roads for kilometres and have to concentrate on the easiest prey to capture: animals domesticated by people. That dramatically reduces their chances of survival.

I feel truly privileged to be invited to a big potlatch in Bella Bella along with Chris and Yoey. This celebration, which used to stretch out over days in the winter months, is put on by an extended family whenever they have a reason to be thankful. The entire community is invited, sumptuously fed and given gifts. The more you can give away, the greater your status in the community. On the tables are pots and pans filled with salmon, halibut, or herring roe – almost unaffordable delicacies on the world market. There are speeches full of gratitude and respect, music and dancing. The celebration begins after the Elders, the wise old people, have taken their places. I note that the young people who otherwise hang out on the roadsides being cool or play basketball to rap music conscientiously lead the Elders to their seats and look after them continuously the entire evening. Although they are growing up in a different age, certain values of communal life remain intact. The young people know what they have in their ancestors. Their culture gave them this tradition.

The dances performed tell stories that have been passed down from the Elders; the musical instruments, the melodies and how to build the drums were relayed to them. The young people look to the experienced ones for advice. So it is in the winter of 2006, when the young people of the village once again gather to party in the forest outside the settlement. As is so often the case, too much alcohol flows. Late in the night, one of the guys decides to go home and leaves his friends. But he's so drunk that he loses his way in the darkness, trips and remains on the ground. It is a clear, icy-cold night. No one notices that he's missing. He falls asleep. If he stays there very long he will freeze. Then he feels something in his face. It is a wolf nudging him gently. Immediately the guy is wide awake, and he just catches a glimpse of the animal slowly withdrawing back into the darkness. The young man runs home quickly and tells his story to the Elders. He wants to know from them what it means. They say simply: "You are Wolf clan. He saved you from dying."

At that same time, I am home in Austria for Christmas. Although it's quite late already, I want to take a short walk in the forest. As I make my way back along the dark, deserted forest path, I suddenly see an unmoving body face down next to the path. Shocked, I stand still and look around. This is really creepy for me. Is there someone else nearby too? Could this be a trap? I pretend I'm not alone out here and talk loudly with my imaginary companion. Nothing moves. I nudge the body. A quiet groan, then motion. I talk to the person, it's a guy about 15 or 16 years old. I ask him what happened and help him stand up. He smells like alcohol.

In bits and pieces I learn something about his past few hours in town, where he drank one too many at a Christmas party and then decided to walk home through the forest by himself. At some point he tripped, fell down and went to sleep. It's a cold night and his body is already chilled. I take him home with me, sit him down next to the warm tiled stove and make him some hot tea. He begs me to please not say anything to his mom. I promise him. A few days later, though, his mother calls me and thanks me, in tears. He told her about it himself.

When I call Pauline, herself an Elder, to wish her a Merry Christmas, she tells me the story of the young Heiltsuk and his rescue by a wolf. And a chill of déjà vu runs down my back.

I grew up in an ecumenical family. Like almost all children in the countryside, we were baptized and received First Communion. For many years I belonged to the Catholic Children's Movement. Gerhild, Mutti, Uncle Dieter and I played music together informally for several years. We played in the nursing home at Christmastime and were part of the Advent concert in the parish church. Several times I was one of the three magi who processed through town in early January. When we children started to get more serious about sports, we were at various competitions most weekends. Our understanding of being Christian wasn't "go to church." Our churches were more the mountains and nature, our church dome the heavenly sky. My parents taught us human values that hold "the good in people" and "doing the right thing" as the highest good: show respect toward all life and nature, be honest, don't waste anything, stay humble and grateful. Overall, we were pretty good kids.

Even if I am only a spectator at the many festivals and ritual celebrations in the course of the year, I enjoy and cherish them very much. Most of them are perpetuated by the church and the farming community, some for many centuries. Both sustain the traditions, pass them on, and by doing so give people a kind of orientation through the year that tells us both about our own origins and the values of our society. That is the 100 per cent positive aspect of this handing down and continuance of the old traditions. But the world moves faster than it ever has before. We humans have gained so much more knowledge and have gotten ourselves into completely new situations and dilemmas. Today, it is more essential than ever to remain open to change and never lose our curiosity and quest for new insights. Our cultural values are the product of our responses to what we know, and are therefore also subject to continuous change.

In the time since the last wolf was eradicated from Central Europe, we have learned a great deal about this animal in other parts of the world, in particular through direct observation and scientific research. And we have realized that the wolf definitely has a positive, useful and very important role. It is up to us to bring our actions into line with current knowledge.

The ranchers now living in western North America are descendants of the Europeans of the 18th and 19th centuries who killed off wolves without knowing anything more about them than that they kill domesticated animals. Even today, most people are not aware of the abundance of new information about wolves and the entire ecosystem in which they – along with humans and others – live. They continue to behave as was customary two hundred years ago.

In Central Europe the situation is no better. Making the effort to learn the latest about wolves was hardly a topic until recently, because wolves were practically extinct. But now that wolves are making inroads and resettling their former territory, we should really endeavour to be familiar with current information about them, and at the same time to take up the traditions we once practised when the wolf was still our neighbour. We have forgotten how to deal with wolves, but in other regions of Europe, where wolves survived and were always present, people continue to use the traditional protective measures – such as shepherding, using dogs to protect flocks, fencing in or corralling domesticated animals – and accept them as a normal part of raising livestock. And they do it in a constructive way, not one that is destructive for the wolves.

Farmers in modern Europe are under immense pressure. They have to feed a growing population, but they earn less and less money for their production. They are financially supported by all kinds of subsidies, but at the same time, it is tempting to make a quick buck by selling land or switching to tourism. Yesterday they milked cows; today they milk tourists. They pose as models advertising our intact environment and healthy food, "On my honour." They are identified as stewards of the land, yet at the same time, chemical fertilizers and spray pesticides that supposedly increase productivity are enticing. Their families are repositories of an incredible amount of traditional knowledge that is often no longer current and not in demand anymore. Farmers thus perform a balancing act between tradition and modernity that is understandably overwhelming for some.

TEK is shorthand for traditional ecological knowledge, the name given to the knowledge of Aboriginal peoples gained over thousands of years. More and more scientists are integrating this traditional knowledge into modern research projects. Aboriginal people are brought on board in order to help scientists gain deeper insight into local and regional activities. In Canada there are many interview projects in which young Aboriginal people ask their Elders questions; through them, TEK is being written down for the first time in their history. It is a race against time, because with every Elder who dies, a unique bit of information can disappear forever. Much has already been irretrievably lost, as is true of many Native languages. Extinguished forever.

Chester is our bearer of the TEK of the Heiltsuk Nation. In addition to natural history, he knows the waters and safe routes for boats; he knows where the "old village sites" are, recognizing by certain signs, such as special patterns of trees or topographical characteristics, where an entire settlement of his ancestors once stood. He shows us lots of "culturally modified trees," ones that were used to make useful things like canoes or Heiltsuk clothing but still live and grow. He leads us to pictographs, ancient rock drawings in red ochre on rock faces sheltered from the weather that continue to transmit their messages to boat passengers who have a sharp eye and as fabulous a guide as Chester. I am always enchanted when he shows us yet another new rock painting, often peering down at us from an overhang, larger than life-sized. How on Earth did the artist climb up there?

It is estimated that more than twenty thousand people once lived here in the coastal forest region, before changes in the climate and the introduction of new diseases drastically reduced the population. I believe these numbers immediately, even if the rainforest has reclaimed the formerly settled areas. When we are out with Lone Wolf, he shows us signs of an earlier, highly developed culture in so many bays and beaches.

Especially interesting for us are the "fish traps," stone walls that were built in the intertidal zone of an estuary. Fish that swam into these during high tide were caught behind the wall when the sea level sank again, and they could easily be gathered. In places where there is such a long tradition of fishing, chances are also good of finding our anglers: wolves, we hear multiple times, are still there today where earlier their kin, the Heiltsuk people, once lived. Interestingly, we find a disproportionate number of wolf dens in places where settlements used to be. With Western logic, we say that these areas are easier to travel through because they were cleared and located in sheltered places and were built near sources of fresh water – all things that also benefit the wolves. Lone Wolf's explanation of it: "They are looking for their ancestors."

Western logic with the additional dimension of the First Peoples' TEK and spiritual background probably comes closest to the truth.

NEWS
SUMMER 2001

I hear a sharp "wuff," and then a second one. Wolves seldom bark. When they do, we are already too close. They use it mainly as a warning signal. This is what happens when filmmaker Twyla and I finally decide to make ourselves known to the wolves. For hours we have been sitting behind a bush at an estuary, observing the pack as they fish for salmon. On a tip from Chester, we hid ourselves there even before the animals came out of the forest for the day. The river immediately became the focus of their attention, and so we have remained undiscovered. Now, however, it's getting dark fast and Twyla and I have a little problem. We are stuck here and the *Tilsup* is anchored out there in the bay, and between us, six unsuspecting wolves are catching salmon. And we can hardly see a thing. The last light is reflected in the water of the ocean and the river and gives us only a few points of reference. For a long time, we hoped the animals would finally have their fill and withdraw to the forest. But that doesn't happen. They give no indication of leaving and continue to fish and camp out. And so – because we don't have any other choice – we decide to make ourselves known. We stand up slowly, without any sudden movements, and talk to each other in a calm tone. Immediately, even the juiciest salmon is of no interest, and all pairs of amber eyes stare at us. "Wuff." Excited splashing in the river; I can still just make out the silhouettes of the lighter wolves, but the darker ones are swallowed in the darkness. "Wuff." It's coming closer. I feel a certain anxiety and feel it gathering in Twyla, too. She is counting on me. I'm her guide and am responsible for her. So I slowly pull the pepper spray out of my bag and release the safety. This is the first and only time I have ever held pepper spray at the ready in the presence of wolves. It's an extreme situation, because we were not forthright with the wolves, but instead kept ourselves hidden, and now – in the darkness – surprised them. They see much better than we do by so little light, however, and surely notice our uncertainty as we move through the darkness toward the beach. As shy and generally well-disposed as wolves are toward people, they get bolder and friskier as night falls. And so I talk into the night, knowing that pricked-up wolf ears are listening. I explain to them what we plan to do, and I apologize for the disturbance. I know that if these animals sense respect and a certain calmness and trust, they will interpret that as strength, and that soothes them. Nonetheless, I'm still very nervous. We don't see the black wolf, but we hear him near us barking very angrily. We continue moving straight toward the beach, where I can finally make radio contact with JM. The wolves have communicated unmistakably that they don't think much of our game of hide and seek.

I'm aware that my feel for this kind of message becomes more and more finely tuned over the course of years in the wilderness, and I note how much more I can decipher from these – sometimes only very subtle – bits of information. The sudden warning cry of a squirrel in a calm, isolated lagoon sounds like a jet plane; or a fine hair on a small branch waving gently in the breeze can tell me an entire story. Over the years, everything around me has become more vivid, because I am in continual, intense exchange with my surroundings.

After my return to civilization, I always get sweaty palms when I have to call strangers on the phone. I don't like it at all; I'm missing all the important information about my conversation partner, information that a voice alone can't provide. I am a visual learner, have to see everything new for myself to be able to store it. I remember foreign words or bird songs poorly after hearing them, or not at all. I need images to go with the sounds. That probably explains why I always have to go out into the three-dimensional world. My spatial perception was always excellent; maybe my papa, who was an excellent civil engineer, gave me a few good genes for that. I once wanted to be an architect, go to Africa some day and build water supply systems for the people there. That's why I was the only girl in my class in the upper grades of high school who, when forced to choose, decided to take descriptive geometry instead of biology. I still took the Matura exam in biology; it was always my favourite subject – taught by my favourite teacher.

My good spatial orientation not only helped me in the wilderness, it also deeply influenced my philosophy of life: depending on your perspective, the same thing can look very different. And to come to a common denominator, you have to either change your point of view or turn the thing until it fits the description of other observers. You might call that building bridges. Only then can a reciprocal exchange of information take place.

Even if I don't like to reach for the phone myself, I've received many of the most decisive messages of my life by telephone: when the phone rang in the summer of 1993 and Franz Puckl invited me to take part in the World Trophy, the world championship in mountain running; in summer 2000 when Carolyn Callaghan interviewed me by phone from the Canadian Rockies, which brought me to Canada for the Central Rockies Wolf Project three months later; when I picked up the receiver in the little bunkhouse in Kootenay National Park in winter 2001 to hear Lyle Wilson, whose phone number I had found on Murphy's collar. When in the fall of 2004 Heinz von Matthey from ZDF was on the other end of the line with a simple question: "Are you interested in making a film about your work with the coastal wolves?" And finally, when the phone rang in spring of 2011 and Heike Hermann introduced herself: "I saw the film about you and the wolves. I am an editor for a large German publishing group. I want to ask if you have time and desire to write a book." All these requests had an enormous influence on the course of my life because I always said "YES!"

But the most important calls of all were ones I had to make: first the daily calls home in the late summer of 1999, when I made a month-long road trip through the western part of Canada and saw traces of wild wolves for the first time – while at home Papa was already failing; later, when I had to call Mutti at home in Austria from Canada after being diagnosed with cancer; and since then, the calls I make with a racing heartbeat and a deep breath after every checkup to hear the news from the doctor, always profound: "Everything okay?" – "Okay!" And then, once again, I feel how enormous the stone is that lifts from my shoulders in that moment. There are things one never gets used to hearing. They change lives forever.

WOLF SPIRIT 3
OCTOBER 2005

After I've had several days of intense headaches, Phil finally convinces me to see a doctor. Reluctantly, I follow his advice. He comes with me. The doctor does a CT scan of my head; the hospital in Canmore just got this piece of equipment recently. We go get some coffee while we wait for the results. It would be the last carefree coffee for a long time.

Back in the hospital, the young doctor enters the room and hangs a black-and-white image on the light board. "At least now we know why you have these headaches. Gudrun, this, here, is a brain tumour..." I don't hear anything else. I pass out and fall into Phil's arms. Through a veil of shock and the feeling I'm having a nightmare, I still hear that I should get my things immediately and go to the bigger Foothills Hospital in Calgary. They are already waiting for me. Paralyzed by the news, I call my mom in Austria: "Mutti, please sit down. I have a brain tumour. I'll have surgery next week." Then Lyle. "Gudrun, I'm coming right over to Canmore and I'll take Nahanni with me to Nipika. Don't worry about a thing," he stammers. I pack some things while Phil makes a few phone calls. When I lock the door behind me, a strange feeling of a new beginning washes over me. I don't know if or when I will open this door again. And as we slowly leave the mountains behind us and they grow smaller and smaller on the horizon, I make a silent wish that they will patiently wait for me. I want to come back home to this place.

NAHANNI
AUTUMN 2002

I happen to see her in a yard in the hamlet of Edgewater, playing with her brother. Not anticipating this chance meeting, I am still completely enchanted by my first glimpse of her. Before reason can interfere, I'm already ringing the doorbell. A young guy opens the door.

"Yes?" he asks, somewhat surprised.

"I saw the puppy in your yard. Is it by chance looking for a home?"

"Come on in."

"Thanks. I was just on my way to see friends…" At that moment, two full-grown dogs bound toward me and greet me enthusiastically.

"These are the parents, belong to me and my girlfriend. The puppy and the eight others in the litter were a climbing accident."

"A what?"

"Well, Anna and I were hanging on a vertical face in a crag when we saw our two dogs making puppies. By the time we were on the ground again, it was too late." I have to chuckle. "But we live with our dogs and for our dogs. The little one, well, we've already promised her to someone in Toronto."

"Toronto?"

The young man may have read the concern in my facial expression as I give him my phone number with the parting request, "Call me if you should change your mind."

A few days later I am flying to the coastal rainforest of Bella Bella again for research work during the fall salmon run. On a mild late-summer evening I get a call from Edgewater. "Gudrun, we changed our minds. We think our little girl will have a better life with you and your lifestyle than in a big city. You can have her."

I'm standing on the deck of our sugar shack looking into the fading evening sky. The ocean is very calm. But I can feel a huge wave of joy surging over me. I have a dog again! Someone I can experience life with, and share adventures, joys and sorrows.

Three weeks later our research in the coastal rainforest is complete for the season. The Inside Passage ferry brings us southward again, into civilization, to Vancouver Island. And once again, after weeks of simplicity and living close to nature, we are overwhelmed by every aspect of civilization, by the many people with their houses, utility poles, fences, fields, roads and cars.

Car? I need a car! I have a dog now, and in spite of the name, Greyhound buses aren't going to work for me anymore as my main means of transportation. So it's time to look for a car as soon as I arrive in Victoria. I meet Danny, my former teammate from Kootenay National Park, who lives in Victoria now and, in addition to everything else, naturally, is also an expert in cars. I'm quite aware that it would be a preprogrammed disaster for me as a young, blonde woman with a foreign accent and limited budget to buy a used car on my own.

Three days later, and with Danny's blessing, I am the proud owner of a 1987 four-wheel-drive Toyota 4Runner with 250,000 kilometres on the speedometer. I set off to pick up Nahanni, a thousand kilometres away in Edgewater. Nahanni – that will be her name, my little one, my new partner, hopefully for many, many years.

It's November and bitter cold. And I can't close my electric window all the way; I stuff the opening with a piece of fabric, but there's an icy wind blowing into the car. I spend the night in my rolling palace in the parking lot of a service station; everything is frozen, including me. Shortly before reaching my destination, the oil light goes on, again. At a gas station in Golden comes the devastating news: the oil pan is cracked, the oil is leaking and sticking to everything under the hood. But if I drive carefully and always keep two or three containers of oil in the car, I should make it, the mechanic assures me. Your word in God's ear, I think, and end my drive late at night in the bunkhouse of Kootenay National Park. And then – finally – the next day I can pick up my Nahanni.

Nahanni, the name of a she-wolf in one of my favourite novels, *In the Shadow of the Rainbow*, is a Cree word that means something like "the people far away on the other side of the river." There is also a national park in the Northwest Territories named after the river that is the main reason for the heavily protected status of that region: the Nahanni River. It is my life's dream to paddle on this river. Nahanni, my future loyal companion, is supposed to remind me of my dream so it doesn't slip away.

Nahanni: the name is almost a short melody, playful and affectionate. And my Nahanni becomes the personification of this beautiful word. She's a head-turner in the dog world, full of grace and pride, and at the same time has this wild, natural core that lets her independence and urge to lead shine through: a husky–shepherd mix with an unknown portion of wolf. The fact is, she feels very much at home in the wilderness, is always completely attentive to her wild surroundings, secure and self-confident in nature, somewhat shy and keeps her distance around too many people, but is extremely friendly with strangers. From the moment she bestows her trust in someone, they will always be greeted with fierce tail wagging and howling. The powerful beats of her tail are definitely the more dangerous end of Nahanni.

As I drive back to the bunkhouse that evening with my friend Piia and the four-month-old dog bundled on her lap, a pack of seven wolves appears in the headlights of my 4Runner (yes, it's still running!) and welcomes Nahanni to her new world. On this drive she surely doesn't suspect it yet, but in the coming seven years she will encounter quite a few wolves at my side. Nahanni is a part of me. And I think I am a part of her.

Night Shift

FOOTHILLS

LIGHT ON THE HORIZON
SPRING 2005

Charles is a genuine bushman. Calmly, with an attentive look in his dark eyes and a mischievous smile, he sits in his old pickup truck and leans out of the open window. "Gudy, I've got a little job for you again. Do you want to help me with night guarding down in the Whaleback area? The U Ranch had a couple of wolf attacks on their herd of young cattle. They're Willow Creek wolves – I put a transmitter on one of them. We have to keep them away from the herd, otherwise they'll shoot them. I kept watch there the past three nights but have to go to Calgary for a few days. Can you spell me?"

Charles is not a man of big words but very much one of big deeds. With infinite patience and often without pay, he has worked for decades for the preservation of the wolf population in southwest Alberta. It's a hot spot for the wolves who live there. This region is the true Wild West, the beauty of the landscape unsurpassed: out of the perfectly flat horizon in the east, the foothills of the seemingly endless prairie roll toward the Rocky Mountains. The closer you get to the mountains, the more the ground undulates and buckles upward. The grass growth on the plains gives way to aspens, with bushy undergrowth, especially along the unfettered, meandering brooks and rivers. Farther to the west, the first conifers gradually replace the deciduous trees, and the forest gets thicker and stretches into higher elevations until it runs into its limits on the steep, sparse mountainsides. The peaks greet the flatlands with gleaming white snow most of the year. This mosaic of varying altitudes and climate conditions generates different plant communities and ecosystems, diverse habitats that provide a suitable home, the necessary habitat, for almost every kind of animal in North America.

And precisely in this narrow north–south strip of land, known as the foothills, is where the most fertile pastures for cattle are located. One ranch abuts the next; with their gigantic grazing lands, the ranches deliver the classic setting for Western movies. And yes, they exist there, the Clint Eastwood types, the range riders, the cowboys of our Western fantasies. Their wear hats of the same name, a bandana, of course jeans, boots to complement the outfit, and – most important in the scene – the most conspicuous belt buckle possible. They are walking clichés who traverse the land with their horses and herding dogs, checking the fences and sometimes driving the herds long distances to new pastures. This is Chinook Country. The chinook is a warm and dry wind that races down the eastern flank of the Rockies and can transform the infamous icy-cold temperatures of the winter prairie into T-shirt weather. And it is so strong that the locals tell stories of flying cows; they are proud to live in Chinook Country. Today, Canada's largest wind power station is located there.

The climate is dry in the weather shadow of the Rocky Mountains, the grassy areas are sparse, the herds large – one cannot make a comparison between the population of bovines on a Chinook Country ranch and the ubiquitous couple of cows kept by people throughout the alpine countries. Between 1,500 and 2,000 head are normal for a southern Alberta herd. That's why the cattle need enormous rangelands and spend most of the time far away from human infrastructure and human protection. They graze, rest and deliver their calves out there, typically alone in the wilderness. And at exactly the time when hungry bears are waking up from their hibernation and urgently need protein, exactly when the wolves are also bearing their young, and just when the elk herds, emaciated from the winter, are trying to rebuild their strength, precisely on the same pastures where the cattle and their newborns are. And with the wild hoofed animals come all their predators, including cougars.

It is April and peak season in ranch country. And to make matters even more complicated, one more species comes into play: human beings. As if there weren't enough complex eat-and-be-eaten relationships here, people now get involved, with their particular demands and valuations, including two opposing points of view. On the one side are the defenders of their cattle, and that is meant in the most literal way possible. They often behave in true Wild West manner: they shoot at almost everything that moves, set traps, and don't hold back from even the most detestable of all defensive methods, namely setting out poisonous bait. The other side has a name and a face for the next four nights: mine. I am working on behalf of the Southern Alberta Cattle Commission (sacc), a co-operation of governmental organizations, cattle ranchers, scientists and environmental agencies whose goal is to reduce the killing of domesticated animals by wolves, and thereby also reduce the uncontrolled murder of wolves. And to do so in a non-lethal way, without any bloodshed. We want to protect the herds too, but with more modern and socially acceptable methods. With very idealistic, or even crazy methods. Carried out by crazy people.

I accept Charles's offer. I love his self-contained personality, admire his knowledge and understand his language. We get along very well. Charles speaks many languages: that of nature and the wild animals, and that of the ranchers and cowboys. He understands all sides and everyone understands him – the best starting point from which to accomplish something in this territory. Only in the lecture halls is he uncomfortable, and acquiring sponsors is a foreign concept for him. So the work in southwest Alberta is more of a labour of love for him. He doesn't earn any money for it. Instead, he earns his living as one of the most sought-after grizzly bear trappers for large research projects in northern Canada. He used to work in the oil fields, dirty work that he doesn't like to talk about. Now he explains to me, referring to an old, crinkled map, where I should look after the herds of young animals for the next few nights. The map isn't very illuminating, but Charles's concentration on the essentials is enough of a guidepost. "Here's the telemetry set. And the light flares. Let me know when you're outside again. Good luck."

"Na, Nahanni? Are you ready? I certainly wouldn't be involved in this madness without you!" Nahanni looks out the window and doesn't say anything. Nahanni is three years old and already used to quite a lot with me. But what lies in wait for us in the coming days and nights will push both of us beyond our comfort zones. I turn in to the driveway of the U Ranch and pass through the great wooden archway from which a sun-bleached steer skull hangs. Five hundred metres farther, the rancher greets me with a brief tip of his cowboy hat. He is just getting the all-terrain vehicle (ATV) ready for me. Then he explains again how to find the right herd, and I get another "Good luck" along the way, this time along with a look of disbelief and a light shake of the head. He is one of the few co-operative cattle owners who allow us to use our various measures to keep wolves away on his property. He lets us do it but without really actively supporting our ideas. The entire cowboy culture here is male, more male-oriented than almost any other group in society. Nonetheless – or maybe because of it – my experience with cowboys is that they are gentlemen if you treat them with full respect. They are allergic to being patronized, whether by government or clever students who have no practical experience. A sticker that sums up their values can be found on the bumpers of more than a few of the area's pickup trucks: "NO gun control, NO wheat pool, NO wolves."

I gratefully take over the ATV and drive slowly into the rolling landscape, Nahanni running and panting alongside the truck. Soon I don't see any indications of human presence, just a landscape that organizes itself and constantly renews itself. A feeling of harmony comes over me. If I ever have the chance to choose anywhere in the world at which to live in a little log cabin, it would be right here.

Now I see the herds, peacefully grazing in a little river valley, in a grove of young aspens. I set up my tent, the place where I will sleep during the day. Even before I pull the last pieces of the tent out of the bag, I am surrounded by lots of big, curious, dark eyes as large as saucers, and Nahanni is in full swing keeping the young cows away. With no success. I hope the bear-proof food box will also keep curious calves from helping themselves to my supplies.

For the night watch, Nahanni and I climb onto a little rise. With a sleeping bag, a headlamp, a good book, and most important a telemetry setup, bear spray and light flares. I have good signal reception here.

Slowly it gets dark, and a night without moonlight spreads itself across the land. Apart from the small radius of my little headlamp, it is pitch black. At the foot of the hill, I think I can hear the cows chewing their cud. In the land of bears, cougars, wolves and coyotes, there are noises everywhere. Every 20 minutes I turn on the telemetry device, hold the antenna up into the black night and listen for the distinctive "peep peep peep" of the radio transmitter on the neck of a wolf in the local pack. Everything is calm; only the wind is beginning to pick up. It increases the rustling all around me. Is it only the wind? Or a mouse or a cow? A coyote, a cougar or a bear? Each sound could be caused by any of those. Why did I agree to take on this job, again? Nahanni's senses are reeling; she continually turns her ears in every direction, attentively lifts her nose into the wind and tries to scan the darkness. She is tense. She is scared, too. Probably more out of empathy with me than fear for herself; she has already chased wolves and young grizzly bears away from me. The night is long, but it does come to an end without anything happening. At 4:00 am, a thin, bluish haze of light to the east heralds the morning, and a lone bird's call releases us from the deep night. Ironically, the orange-yellow strip of artificial light coming from the oil metropolis of Calgary, more than 150 kilometres away, eases my loneliness somewhat. Inwardly, I breathe a deep sigh of relief. If something were to approach the cattle at this point, I could at least see its outline. These nights leave behind an intense impression: how helpless and vulnerable I feel when I can't see. The dawn reconciles us with the challenges of the wilderness. And after breakfast, we both sleep until the brindled clowns find us again. Later in the day, Nahanni and I stroll through the hills dotted with shrubs and climb a little hill.

I can make out two vegetation corridors in the landscape that could definitely serve as wolf trails. Will the wolves actually use them the next night? As darkness falls, we take up our position on the "signal hill" again. The night begins like the previous one. I am alert and full of doubt about my life philosophy, or rather the age I'd like to attain: 96 and healthy. That being so, there can't be too many more nights like this one. At some point, I routinely raise the antenna and immediately freeze. "Peep peep peep" rings out, and loudly. They are on the move. Somewhere out there in the jet-black night. They are coming from the more densely forested regions in the northwest. I hear the cattle mooing. Nahanni jumps up, and I pack my light flares, bear spray and telemetry antenna. I can hardly see where I'm going, Down, just down, and faster than reasonable thoughts can catch up to me. Taking the shortest route to the ATV. Even before I start the engine, I turn on the blinding high beams to scare off the wolves, and probably to give me a little sense of security, too. The signal tells me the wolves are already in the shallow depression where the cattle are gathered. The mooing is getting more agitated; the animals seem to sense danger. I don't want the herd to disperse, so I leave the ATV where it is and walk a ways on foot. I light one of the flares in the direction the signal is coming from, and a few moments later, a second one. I check the telemetry signal again. Now it's a little farther away and on the other side of the herd. Slowly I walk back to the ATV, continuously checking the movements of the tagged she-wolf. She retreats back over the rise. I nod at Nahanni deep in thought, fully aware that I wouldn't make it through all of this without her. Sleep is the last thing on our minds for the rest of the night, and in the morning the cows find us especially sleepy.

By daybreak the world looks lovely again, and the nocturnal threat has become as unreal as a bad dream. And yet I know that I may have to go through the whole thing again in a few hours. Sometimes it truly would be better if we had no idea what the immediate future would bring.

The danger of an invisible foe is nightmarish, even if it's wolves, whose behaviour I am familiar with. But it's a deeply rooted, primitive fear of the dark, paired with the archaic human memory of potentially dangerous predators and the solitude of the night. And I have already experienced myself, on the Pacific Coast, that wolves behave more boldly at night than during the daylight. They come closer, bark and even snarl. So my psyche has quite a lot to process. In search of some normality, I drive about 40 kilometres to the nearest town, Blairmore, for a late breakfast. I feel protected in the small, colourful café, and ponder what all I could still order to postpone the drive back. I quietly imagine what little secrets the people around me are carrying with them, and what they plan to do when night falls. Then I'm back in the tent in the aspen grove. Everything is just as I left it, as if I never left, and yet the time in between was a little vacation for my soul. I'm not looking forward to the night, but it mercilessly presses its dark mass over the landscape. The grass at our checkpoint on Signal Hill is still trampled from the previous nights. Nahanni immediately curls up in her spot beneath the overhanging branches of a small, wind-stunted digger pine. The tree is living testament to the power of the chinook, which tests the flexibility of everything living in the region, again and again. I read my book; it helps me maintain the illusion that I'm actually somewhere else. Until the signal suddenly starts up again. The wolves are back. With a sigh, I peel myself out of my sleeping bag. Nahanni's expression doesn't match her upright, energetic body position at all. She is just doing her duty as a dog, but she doesn't feel comfortable at all in this situation. "Me either, Nahanni. Me either."

The night is just as black as the previous one, and inwardly I'm also in a kind of black hole. In this role, I protect the wolves by chasing them away. The bizarre logic of people. Everything un-folds just as stressfully as it did almost exactly 24 hours ago. Wolves are a species with traditions and routines. If you want to change their behaviour, then these routines must be energetically broken. That takes time and requires repetition. And you have to know what you're doing. Lots of ranchers still follow the no-win strategy of the "three S's:" shoot, shovel and shut up. In so doing, they ig-nore the fundamental biology of the wolves. If you randomly shoot at a pack and murder random wolves, the entire, complex social structure of the pack is constantly subjected to disruptions. And a pack is one thing above all others: a well-coordinated hunting team in which each individual uses his or her strengths to achieve the common goal, namely capturing prey.

Each member of the group is aware of the role of the other, what he does especially well and how he behaves. A high degree of co-operation and mutual trust, as well as quick, efficient deci-sions taking into account more their own behaviour, and excellent communication, are absolutely necessary during every hunt if it is to be successful. So it is typically the lighter, faster females who chase the prey before the more powerful males attack. In addition, there are wolves in the pack that function as "clowns," distract-ing an intended quarry, for example, or defusing mounting ten-sions within the family with their easygoing antics. And the young wolves observe and learn from the older ones. The individual ani-mals need enough experience and thus time to fit into their roles and to practise for their part in the teamwork. If this highly co-op-erative social fabric is disturbed again and again by the shooting of individual members, in some cases the shooter may cause the exact opposite of what he intended. Instead of keeping the wolves away from his domesticated animals, he now forces them to turn their attention to easier prey, i.e., livestock, because he has com-promised their hunting efficiency. To successfully communicate these connections takes a lot of convincing. All too often, there is a lack of willingness to accept knowledge that comes from outside, especially if it might shatter old, firmly fixed opinions. Progress toward people becoming more relaxed with what is apparently un-controllable will always be made in small steps.

SACC hasn't reached this goal yet, and that's why Nahanni and I have another night ahead of us, which proceeds in a similarly anxious way as the previous ones. This time, though, the wolves come but keep a comforting distance from the pasture. Nonetheless, I want to let them know once and for all that they will be better off finding a fresh elk calf in the forest than to attack the livestock, not to mention the better nutritional value of wild game. So once again I shoot off several loud flares.

Around 4:00 am I just want to hug the reliable glimmer of first light. The dawn is approaching, and I pack up my tent site faster than ever. "The operation was a success – all the patients are still alive!" For now, at least.

I meet Charles and hand over the telemetry equipment. How did it go? "Well, um…" Would I have time again next weekend? "No, I'm sorry I can't, already have something very important going on…"

Ever since humans began keeping animals for their own needs, our relationship with large predators has changed drastically, and for the worse. The wolf has suffered more than any other as a result of our ancestors' new lifestyle; the creature that used to be seen as a model of social life and communal hunting became a hated killer of domesticated animals. Then, as today, unfortunately, people have made an impact on almost all populations of wolves around the world with devastating force, with the goal of completely eradicating these – from the perspective of livestock owners – useless animals. The people found allies in hunters, who also didn't want to accept the natural competition of wolves and other large predators in their search for hoofed animals. And more often than not, livestock owners and hunters are one and the same person anyway.

Even today, almost all ranchers in the Wild West still have a gun in tow, next to them in their pickup trucks or on horseback. Everything with four legs and fur is shot at. Wolves and coyotes are hit the hardest. The bounty paid by the government for every predator killed was an additional incentive, until this practice was discontinued due to a lack of wolves. But in Alberta, bounties are still paid for coyotes. This official practice conveys that these animals not only serve no useful purpose, but should be actively cleared out. Why do people think they know what belongs where, what's good and what's bad? Is it arrogance, or only helplessness? Unfortunately, even today, far too many people continue to believe that problems can be solved through the use of force. The way a society treats its animals, especially the challenging animals – which large predators simply are – is a striking detail that gives an indication how peaceful, creative, generous and tolerant a society is as a whole. It is an indicator that has nothing to do with the usual measures of wealth. On the contrary: Canada, like the USA or the Scandinavian countries, is among the richest countries on Earth. And yet, all of these nations are intolerant of wolves. Even in the 21st century, in the southwest of Alberta, a wolf can be shot without a licence and without a "bag limit," i.e., in unlimited numbers, captured in traps or even killed by poisoning. With this legal tailwind, the ranchers have free run to do what they want with wolves, and often enough they use violence.

As of this writing, according to Alberta's hunting regulations, landowners and livestock owners may shoot wolves without a licence and at any time throughout the year, on their own property or leased grazing lands, as well as on any lands in an 8-kilometre radius around them. There is no precondition that a wolf has killed anything. All other Canadian residents may shoot a timber wolf during the big-game season without a licence. The big-game season typically begins on September 1 and lasts until May 31 or June 15 of the following year (so nine or more months of a year). Non-resident hunters need a licence, which costs a mere $12.40.

The early morning light on the horizon thus takes on a new meaning for me. Although I am incredibly relieved to see it after the nerve-wracking night watches, I know that for the wolves in Alberta, it's the starting shot for a new day full of dangers.

ICY
NOVEMBER 2003

It's coming straight at me. In the headlights of our ramshackle, blue, government-issue car, I see the big lights and the typical row of lights above the driver's cabin racing toward us. A huge truck. I stare at Renee. She is sitting behind the steering wheel, still relatively relaxed. "Are you crazy??" I scream at her. "RIGHT! We drive on the RIGHT side here in Canada!" At the last second, she yanks the steering wheel and the truck thunders past us. "Oh, God, Renee, that was close," I stammer.

"It's a habit ... sorry, have to get used to that," is the sheepish answer of the small, boisterous Australian. *Well, do it soon*, I think. We still have more than a hundred kilometres to go to the cabin at Highwood Pass. It's November and a fierce snowstorm is blowing around our car. Renee is driving on, in and through snow for the first time in her life. And I am deeply regretting my idea to offer her this crash course in "driving in winter conditions for newly arrived Australians." The snowflakes fly against the windshield like stars in the dark universe.

At some point we arrive at our shack at Highwood Junction. It's one of those corrugated-sheet-metal rectangles in which the lightweight US-American "trailer trash" television comedies take place: nothing in it is genuine, everything is a rip-off. This will be our abode for the coming week, until the last calves are taken from the pastures. Then they'll be sent to terrible mass-production facilities known as feedlots, where they'll be fattened and then slaughtered. I eat very little meat, but here in this region I sometimes treat myself to a juicy steak; something equivalent just doesn't exist in Europe. I tell myself I've contributed a little bit to it, namely by protecting herds of young cattle that have already been assailed on the pastures from further wolf attacks in these last few weeks.

For the wolves, this is a critical time of year. By now, the deer born this year are just as difficult to hunt as the mature animals. And while their own wolf pups are already part of the hunting party, they are only in the first stages of learning. But the young ones already have a wolf's appetite and hunger. In these weeks, all these factors lead the wolves to attack young cattle that they haven't paid any attention to all summer. The herds, far from civilization on the seemingly endless, arid fields of grass, need protection now. Especially during the night and in the early morning hours: the time of the wolf.

It's bitterly cold as I steer the truck past the main building of the OH Ranch, briefly let them know I'm on my way out to the herd, and continue rattling along the rough, rocky path toward the forested hills. After we pass the first crest, the ranch already disappears from view. Twice I have to jump out of the truck to open a gate, drive through and then close it again behind me. I pass two herds, each more than five hundred head. The pasture of the herd of young cattle that's already been attacked rises gently toward the forest, with a water trough and scrub in the southern part. Every few days the ranch truck comes and tosses out more hay bales. Only then can you see how big this herd actually is, because then they all run to the same place to get the juiciest parts of the feed. The rest of the time, they're distributed over an enormous area during daylight hours. I usually drive into the fields about an hour before dusk so I can still get an overview of where the animals are. Then I look for a good place to spend the night in the cab of the truck. On the passenger seat next to me is a huge spotlight.

Night settles over the land, and soon I hear nothing but an occasional moo here and there. At irregular intervals I turn on the spotlight and slowly scan the area around the cows. The powerful beam reaches almost a kilometre. In the light I note that the cows have huddled together. They feel their vulnerability; they have already experienced it: the wolves come into the pasture and take one of them. Since the first wolf attack, the rancher has added a full-grown longhorn to the herd. At night, she is their centre. The young animals instinctively look to the old, watchful cow for protection. And a cluster of animals crowded together makes it harder for the wolves; they will only take ones they can recognize as individual animals and single out. And they especially need animals that lose their cool and start running – that behaviour unleashes the wolves' hunting instinct. We lovingly call the herd of young cattle "the clowns" because they are funny, but also because they often start to run without any recognizable reason or destination. The longhorn is a kind of beacon for all of them, providing them with orientation and a sense of security. Adding her was a good move on the rancher's part.

The wolves, nonetheless, try approaching the herd again and again. They've had success before, which motivates them to repeat their attacks on young cows. To discourage the wolves, I lean on the horn. A long, drawn-out "beeeeeeeeeep" penetrates the night and echoes in the darkness. Afterward the silence is even more intense, almost sinister. And so the night passes. By dawn it is icy cold in the truck. There are a few cookie crumbs next to me, and I'm overcome with paralyzing cold and deep exhaustion. With relief, I turn the key in the ignition, drive a tour around the pasture, and meet both of the ranch riders at the first gate. "Everything was calm tonight." One of them, named Heigh, nods gratefully, turns around to his colleague and continues to ride along the fence. On their daily round, the men check the fence, look after their cattle herds, and at regular intervals drive them to new grazing grounds. I drive to Highwood Station, where Renee is already waiting for me.

"How was it?"

"Nothing special, just long, dark and cold. It's your turn tonight. Take a good book with you, no, better take two." Renee is a phenomenon; she swallows books like an Australian crocodile, at least one *Harry Potter* a day. After just a few days, she had become close friends with the librarian in the nearest village, Longview, about 25 kilometres from our quarters. Full of character, this Longview, a little one-street town with history. Built in classic Western style, with a small hotel that once was painted white and doesn't deserve the name "hotel," even in North America, a gas station, a restaurant, a café that belongs to the popular country singer Ian Tyson, and the aforementioned "library." The library single-handedly, hopelessly, competes against the rural, action-based culture of the place and seems almost exotic.

I'm familiar with lots of local public libraries but not because of their books. They all have free access to the Internet and are thus the gateway to the wider world, to friends and family. In the Highwood trailer, thanks to Renee's persistence, we now have a telephone, and of course we each have a radio set for our field-work. Renee bats her eyes mischievously and laughs. She is always laughing, even when she brushes her teeth. Only once she didn't laugh: when a woodrat, also called a packrat, took up residence in the hollow space inside the walls of her room. That's something you wouldn't wish on your worst enemy: absolute worst-case scenario, a nightmare! Though they are rather cute, these animals stink like nothing else on the planet.

As soon as I return from my night watch, I head for my room at the opposite end of the trailer. I'm drawn there for a morning nap, while Renee explores the surrounding area for a while and then drives to the library again.

At noon, we switch vehicles. Renee takes over the heavy government truck, while I have the old Toyota pickup, model RHET: Rust Holds Everything Together. I had already been stationed at Highwood for two weeks when I gently introduced Renee to the wonderful world of night watches on the day after her arrival. We stuck together the first night, then unanimously decided it would be a wonderful thing to be able to sleep at least every other night. So we alternate shifts.

On normal sleeping days, I hike for hours over the hills and cross open, barren slopes. After the first snowfall, I immediately find fresh wolf and bear tracks; this is the season when, for the first time after the dry summer, you can estimate which kinds of animals are where and in what numbers. Then the snow melts again, leaving patches in the shade, the chinook wind comes and dries everything up again, then new snow falls, and then the sun shines again. At this time of year, the landscape presents itself anew every morning, and the search for tracks is just as varied. It takes a lot of persistence and determination to stubbornly follow a trail that hasn't been perceptible to the human eye for several hundred metres because the ground simply doesn't give any clear information. And still I press on, aware that the wolf did exactly that. Over years and countless kilometres of tracking, a kind of inner eye for following traces develops that begins to lead you; it urges me onward, or has me turn, or makes me stop. Most trackers talk about this feeling that occurs when we allow it to, when we simply walk without a purpose or a goal in mind.

Walking is experiencing a renaissance these days. People call it meditative and soothing; many are even going on pilgrimages. When we walk, we move at the pace our senses are best adapted to; we experience our environment most intensely then. Sometimes I feel the boundaries of my body become unclear when I'm tracking. I register every change of the smell in the air, the surface of the ground, the angle of the blades of grass, and the sounds around me. Many a time I've had the depressing sensation of being something like a spy, an invader who is actually disruptive because I'm carrying around too much intellect, which usually drowns out inner knowledge. Outside is a world that is designed and proceeds according to an inner wisdom that resides in everyone and everything. You can call it what you will. It's best to just allow it to be. Generously. Without judging.

Everything has its place and its significance. At some point in time, we all knew that. Then the age of utilitarianism dawned at the beginning of the 19th century, the ethics of usefulness, and people began to evaluate everything according to the answer to the question, What does it do for me or for society?

Many wild animals, indeed, wilderness itself, were devalued by this approach. For the wolves – after they had already been relentlessly persecuted for centuries – this way of thinking was their undoing. Even today one of the central "incriminations" toward wolves is the question, What good are they to me or my kind? An egocentric worldview. An objective answer to that question has only been possible for half a century, since the first systematic wolf research began, initiated by Adolph Murie in the mid-1940s. He was the first scientist to study wolves in their natural habitat, on Mount McKinley in Alaska. At that time, wolves had already died out in Central Europe, so those Europeans had absolutely no objective information about them. Everything they knew was derived from stories about encounters when wolves came out of the forest to kill domesticated animals. The negative experiences stood in the foreground. These were quickly transformed into abstract legends and stubbornly continue to be perpetuated on the European continent.

The ranchers of the North American West are descendants of those white settlers from Europe who had just celebrated the extinction of the last wolves in the middle of the 19th century in their native countries and immigrated to North America with those values in tow. The second major baggage they brought was their cattle. Their arrival would forever change nature with its native flora and fauna, as well as the lives of Indigenous peoples; Contact would even destroy them. The vast herds of bison, estimated to have been 60 to 70 million strong, were massacred within a few years. At the very last moment, a tiny herd of less than a hundred animals was placed under protection in Montana in one of the most far-sighted private initiatives ever undertaken, and the species was thus saved from complete extinction. All modern bison stem from that herd.

The new arrivals continued their crusade against everything wild, with unbelievable cruelty. Wolves, bison, Aboriginal peoples – they have in common the fate of near extinction. The mountain bison didn't make it; that species is considered officially extinct. The settlers slowly worked their way westward and pushed the "last frontier," the boundary against the wilderness, ahead of them. Because the unfamiliar, the uncontrollable and the unpredictable was always on their minds and in sight, their longing for security was roused. And a sense of security can be achieved in one of two ways: by exerting power over something uncontrollable in order to control it, or by acquiring knowledge about the unfamiliar, thus making it familiar and trusted. The first takes place through aggression, while the second approach requires a lot of time, tolerance and openness for that which is new. In the history of humankind, the first way has surely been chosen most often.

My ways are those of the wolves. Sometimes of a single individual, sometimes of a whole pack that tries again and again to be allowed to live peacefully in its natural environment, tenaciously and sometimes in vain. Of course, this is a worldwide phenomenon that is not limited to any one species. When I'm out tracking, I'm in the moment. I feel myself completely in the here and now, and thoroughly alive. The wolves take me to places I would never have gone otherwise, they show me things I would never have perceived, and they open boundaries for me that I would otherwise never have crossed. They convey a certain single-mindedness, sometimes almost an indifference, toward challenges. They make my life richer.

I turn my attention back to my surroundings. As I was thinking, I've walked a good way farther; I've reached the highest point of the trail and marvel at the view. Wolf spirit – such astonishing nature! And you are a part of it. I have to turn back. Renee is probably already waiting for me to take over. Sometimes it's hard to return to the realm of time.

That evening I'm back out in the field. I can feel the effects of the long hike in my muscles, and I'm fighting sleepiness. Just don't fall asleep, don't fall asleep, don't fall … Suddenly I'm awoken by loud motor sounds. As if hit by a bolt of lightning, I'm immediately wide awake. Here come two pairs of headlights directly toward my truck. Which is parked miles away from any public road in a vast expanse of grazing grounds. Who can it be? It's shortly after 3:00 am. I break out in goosebumps. Oh, lord – right, around 11:00 pm, a couple of hunters who were out with Heigh stopped by; they tried to insist that I join them at the pub in Longview to share a drink to celebrate their successful elk hunt. I told them I was working right then, and they could bring me a beer on their way home.

These guys had clearly already had a few even before their trip to the pub, so I was sure they would forget all about me. Now I regret having said that bit about bringing me a beer. Because at this moment, a group of drunken hunters is staggering toward me in the middle of the night, in the middle of nowhere. I want to start the truck, but it doesn't make a sound. Dammit. I fell asleep with the lights on; the battery is empty. Now I even need their help! The first one is already laying on the horn of his pickup and yanks my door open. Grinning, he pulls a bottle of beer from the side pocket of his denim jacket. I fall back in my seat, take a deep breath and release a disbelieving, "Wow – didn't think you guys…" I don't get any further. With an awkward, move he pulls himself into the cabin of my truck, at the same time pushing me onto the passenger's seat.

"Doesn't start, eh?"

"Empty battery," I mutter.

"Hey, Joe, we need the jumper cables! Toss them over!" In no time, the ranch riders have my truck running again.

I sit with wide-open eyes next to my uninvited chauffeur. "And what now?"

"It's probably best to drive you to our hunting cabin back there in the woods. You must be cold. And have you eaten anything tonight?"

"Well, yeah, I ate something…"

"Too long ago. We'll make you something warm. Hey, Heigh, the lady's hungry – fire up the barbecue!"

When the hunting cabin appears in the headlights, I recognize the bodies of two large animals next to it, hanging with spread legs from a thick, round beam. An elk and a moose, which look gruesome in that condition. Like a gentleman, one of the hunting heroes gives me a hand as I jump down from the truck. Heigh is already heating up the barbecue grill on the small front terrace. Then I see the actual bounty from the pub squirming their way out of the second truck: two bleached-blond cowgirls, wearing jeans tighter than their own skin. Oh no, what have I gotten myself into again? Furtively, I look around for my truck. Should I just take off? It's blocked by the other vehicles.

My dinner is ready. Steak and canned peach preserves. The steak blows my mind, so juicy and perfectly grilled. I note that I was genuinely hungry and throw Heigh a look of appreciation. The ranch rider responds with a question: "Why do you do that?" He means my job on the cattle pastures.

Okay, I think to myself, that was the opening shot, and I can already picture myself hanging next to the two wild animals outside the cabin. And to top everything off, today of all days, I'm wearing the red T-shirt that Lone Wolf gave me a few weeks ago as a parting present when I left the coast. It has a wolf's head on the front. One of those kitschy, romanticized images of a wolf. So I decide to plunge straight ahead and start the first lesson: the facts of wolf biology. Then I explain in simple terms why I do this "crazy" work and try to explain to him that wolves only attack cattle because shooting kills some of their numbers randomly, which hugely interferes with their social structure and their ability to hunt wild prey.

As I talk, I avoid direct references to the current situation of this particular herd and these particular men, who are sitting tightly crowded around a small, battered wooden table with me in the cabin. But I do also talk about agriculture at home in the Alps, various types of Austrian beer, and cross-country skiing. Everyone listens with remarkable respect. Then Heigh starts to talk: "Sorry, Gudrun, but I hate wolves. I kill every one I can get. You know, I'm out there and help the newborn calves plow their way through the deep, heavy spring snow to their mothers to nurse. And then the next day I see the calves standing there with their intestines hanging out. Oh my God, how I hate those damned beasts."

I nod. And start over from the beginning: "Yeah, we don't want either one, dead calves or dead wolves. That's why we're trying to test different, non-lethal methods that are intended to minimize the killing of cattle. Whether that's night watches or putting up fladgery – lines with strips of red cloth hanging from them, which wolves won't cross – or using more barns in cattle farming or cutting back on the hunting of wolves' natural prey, like elk and deer, in areas where cattle herds are affected." It occurs to me that no one at this table has ever given a thought to the wolf, except that it should be eradicated. Thanks to the ever-present fascination that wolves exert on anyone who has at least a little objective information about their social structure, family life, communication or hunting strategies, I, too, have interested listeners.

After a brief silence, someone suddenly says, "Hey, Joe, that's right! That's goddamn right!" I will never forget that exclamation; I carry it in me as a constant spark of hope that is always rekindled when it seems we're talking to brick walls of human prejudices. For me, this outcry represents the ever-present possibility of changing people's minds, the power of mutual respect and building bridges, and the opportunities that come about when we focus on what we have in common instead of what separates us. In the course of my work on behalf of wolves, I have repeatedly experienced similar "Aha!" moments of insight with wolf killers. Often they aren't even antagonistic toward wolves, they just kill wolves out of habit.

The most famous example of this kind of conversion is documented by Aldo Leopold:

> [I]t was a wolf. A half-dozen others, evidently grown pups, sprang from the willows and all joined in a welcoming melee of wagging tails and playful maulings.... In those days we had never heard of passing up a chance to kill a wolf. In a second we were pumping lead into the pack, but with more excitement than accuracy.... When our rifles were empty, the old wolf was down, and a pup was dragging a leg into impassable slide-rocks.
>
> We reached the old wolf in time to watch a fierce green fire dying in her eyes. I realized then, and have known ever since, that there was something new to me in those eyes – something known only to her and to the mountain. I was young then, and full of trigger-itch; I thought that because fewer wolves meant

more deer, that no wolves would mean hunters' paradise. But af-
ter seeing the green fire die, I sensed that neither the wolf nor the
mountain agreed with such a view.

Since then I have lived to see state after state extirpate its
wolves. I have watched the face of many a newly wolfless moun-
tain, and seen the south-facing slopes wrinkle with a maze of
new deer trails. I have seen every edible bush and seedling
browsed, first to anaemic desuetude, and then to death. I have
seen every edible tree defoliated to the height of a saddlehorn.
Such a mountain looks as if someone had given God a new prun-
ing shears, and forbidden Him all other exercise. In the end the
starved bones of the hoped-for deer herd, dead of its own too-
much, bleach with the bones of the dead sage, or molder under
the high-lined junipers.[2]

I'm back in the pasture in time for the sunrise. Everything is
calm. Thank heavens. I wait for the next critical hour to pass, then
start to make my way back toward the Highwood trailer. Tired but
impressed, I'm sitting at the steering wheel when Heigh, already
on his morning patrol of the cattle, rides toward me. He signals
to me that I should stay put. I roll down the window and wait.
"Gudrun, I want to apologize for last night. I was a little bent out
of shape about the whole wolf thing." I smile. At him and inwardly.
The ice has been broken.

COAL
SPRING 2003

Coal has disappeared yet again. This dark wolf is really keeping me
on my toes. He is the champion roamer among our tagged wolves.
Here today, tomorrow almost 80 kilometres farther south. How on

2 Aldo Leopold, *A Sand County Almanac*, accessed July 29, 2015, http://faculty.
ithaca.edu/mismith/docs/environmental/leopold.pdf. Aldo Leopold (1887–
1948) was a US-American forestry scientist, wildlife biologist, hunter and ecol-
ogist. He is considered one of the founders of the environmental protection
movement.

earth does he do that, especially with a paw that's missing a toe? He sacrificed it when he stepped into a foothold trap – he chewed it off so he could continue to live freely. Since then he has roamed along the foothills on the eastern flank of the Rockies. In addition to the night watches south of Kananaskis Country, I try to keep up with Coal during the day. This means refilling my gas tank often.

For months, Coal has been demonstrating to us what a wolf is capable of. For me he is the prime example of a wolf, and he is unfortunately also experiencing the typical story for the wolves in this area: permanently looking for something, constantly on the run. He knows every tree along the foothills, but he has never found a place to call home. I've followed him for hundreds of kilometres without ever seeing him. He is the embodiment of humans' hatred of the uncontrollable; we project our acute discomfort onto him. As soon as he appears, he's already gone again. He corresponds perfectly to the myth of the spectral wolf.

Over the months, I develop a deep feeling of sympathy toward him. Through him I've learned that it's not always necessary to have someone very close and constantly in view in order to build a relationship. I've also learned that it's important to always meet your counterpart with respect, which can be expressed to a wolf with spatial distance. Only then do you get a true picture of him; his tracks are undistorted, the way he determines with his free will.

And it was with Coal, this wolf I so greatly respect and admire, with his adroit cleverness, that I once overstepped that respectful boundary. This remains even today the experience I most regret.

I located his signal in the steep flanks of the Livingstone Range. From the dusty gravel road I'm driving along, I get an excellent bearing. I immediately pull over onto the shoulder, jump out of the car, throw my backpack over my shoulder and walk over the last patches of snow, slowly disappearing under the warm spring sunshine, directly toward the signal. The volume assures me that I'm still far enough away that the wolf won't notice me. But the signal quickly grows louder. I begin to move forward by creeping from cover to cover. Then I come across his trail. Clearly pressed into the snow, it leads diagonally up the steep northern slope. The snow becomes very deep; here the land is covered by a permanent shadow in winter. In places it's so steep that Coal worked his way upward in bounds. Even without a signal, this track would have let me know that it's him: one paw print has three toes. And at regular intervals, I find some blood in it.

I'm up to my hips in snow at some points. It's obvious that this slope is prone to avalanche. Now at the latest I should have turned around, but that only became clear to me after the fact. I know everything I need to know for my monitoring. And Coal is on land that is part of a ranch whose owners are pro-wolf. So he is safe here and should stick around as long as possible. But instead I tramp onward. The steepness of the terrain and the depth of the snow make it impossible to check Coal's signal regularly. Finally, I reach a small grove of dwarf birch trees outside the avalanche channel. The terrain is somewhat flatter here. I catch my breath and take another reading. He is very close, so close that the attenuator, the signal that you only receive in the immediate vicinity of the transmitter, sounds. He must be crouched there in the grove in front of me. All at once my adrenaline level plunges and a sudden, sobering awareness comes to me. I come to my senses. I've been chasing him, urging him on ahead of me. This wolf, the one whose ghost-like quality and endurance in the face of all kinds of dangers I so admire – I hunted down this wolf.

Yet again, in the deep snow and steep terrain, he was forced to demonstrate his will to live and wrote it in the snow with his blood. Suddenly I start to cry, from exhaustion, but especially out of sympathy for Coal. I'm disappointed in myself for not being able to resist the greedy desire to finally see Coal with my own eyes, a desired result that comes at the expense of this wolf that has already been severely persecuted. Now he has to flee one more time. For me, it is a new, singular and sad experience.

I begin to talk with him, slowly apologizing toward the brush in which two attentive ears are hidden. I continue to talk soothingly as I slowly make my retreat. Coal should know that I'm not one of them.

When I reach the car again, I feel the full force of the spring sun. I blink up at the shadowy, cold slope where Coal, the wolf, can now find some peace.

A few months later he is chased for the last time. The pursuit ends fatally for Coal.

SILENCE
WINTER 2002

I still have a little time before I drive out to the fields for night watch, and I haven't looked for the tagged wolves for quite a while. With their extreme roaming, it's like winning the lottery when you catch their signals anyway. But if you don't ever play, you can't win anything at all. So I steer the black pickup truck, its rattles already familiar, northward into Kananaskis Country, a partially protected provincial park system along the eastern flank of the Rocky Mountains. It's also the weekend playground of a million residents of Calgary and its surroundings.

It's late November, cold, and the roads are icy. I drive along the Sheep River. The river meanders freely through its carved-out valley. It generates gravel bars and opens onto meadows where the first crystals of ice sparkle now. This is one of my favourite valleys, as soon as the many day visitors are back in their warm houses in the big city and peace is restored. At this time of year, it's very lonely here. I haven't encountered a single other car. Slowly the daylight is ebbing, too. Somewhere I see a little light shining from a cabin, then nothing. I leave the valley and turn onto Gorge Creek Trail. A narrow, winding gravel road climbs steeply upward. On the left side of the road, a steep, rocky cliff falls away to Sheep Valley far below. The name is apt; this is perfect terrain for the Rocky Mountain bighorn sheep, and it's cougar territory too.

The road levels out and dense forest covers the knoll. Now it leads steeply back down on the north side of the hill. This little road is a valuable shortcut to the Elbow River Valley to the north.

I've seen signs of wolves along this connector several times before. Wolves love a good shortcut too. *Oh, the road is completely covered with ice!* I think, and I shift down into first gear. As I release the clutch, my truck starts to slide. I immediately lose control of the vehicle. It has no traction anymore and doesn't respond at all, except to gravity, which is pulling the truck relentlessly downward. A sharp left curve appears in the headlights. The truck careens to the right. Toward Gorge Creek Canyon. A deep chasm. *Is this it?* shoots through my mind. And at the same time, in absolute desperation, I jerk the steering wheel to the left. At the last second, the vehicle changes course and races toward the brush-covered slope at the left side of the road. There it smashes head-on into the hill with full force. And flips over. It's deathly silent for a moment. Then the cab collapses into itself with a loud crash. I breathe for the first time. Over. It's over. It's completely dark all around me. And quiet. Pressure on my head. I'm hanging head down in the destroyed vehicle. I don't want to look at the rest of me. I don't feel anything yet, no pain, nothing. I just want out, out of there fast, just get away. I climb through the shattered windshield, but first I grab my radio set. That's essential for my survival now. Then I stand on my own two legs next to the truck. Yes, I can stand. I can walk. It's pitch black, cold and absolutely still. Then I look up. You automatically look up when you climb out of an old truck that's lying on its roof and instantly recognizable as totalled. Its four wheels spin in the air, out of place. Like a helpless turtle on its back. And far above I see the stars now. It is a clear, cold night that's only enlivened by the billions of stars. I walk back along the road that was supposed to bring me to the wolves just a short while ago. I have to move immediately. Otherwise I might start to feel pain or to freeze or – worst of all – to think. Again and again I desperately radio for help. "Is anyone out there? Dispatch. Dispatch." The night remains silent. I'm frustrated. I know how far it is to Turner Valley and can't even think about it. Even the Sheep valley is far away and devoid of people. Wait, I stop my own thoughts. There was that light I saw driving in! I've never noticed an inhabited cabin in the valley before, but today I saw a light there. That's where I have to go. I just have to make it that far. I walk. Forward. Into the uncertain darkness.

Now the forest and the night begin to talk. Noises everywhere. I think about the cougars and bears. Especially the cougars. They give me the creeps. I don't know much about them. I've never seen a cougar in the wild, but I am certain that many of them have followed me attentively with their cat eyes. They stalk the way big cats do. From behind. And they're nocturnal. I shiver. I think about the fact that no one knows where I am, and no one will miss me, at least not until noon tomorrow, when I should return to our cabin after my night watch and Renee will be expecting me.

I walk, utterly alone. One step after the other. I don't think about the entire way to the light, just about the next step. It's the most important thing now. It takes me toward the light. Suddenly I have to think about my papa. Very urgently. I have the feeling that he's sitting there in the stars; yes, he's definitely up there. And he's guiding me, in his way. He wasn't one to give up either. He was a calm, tenacious fighter. His journey through his serious illness lasted almost six years, until he exhausted himself. Tomorrow will be the third anniversary of his death. I have to reach the light before I'm exhausted. The cold is merciless. The song that my brother wrote within a few hours of our father's death pops into my head: "Papa, you did it your way..." I sing it for kilometres and hours, again and again. I have something to do. And it isn't even so bad. The darkness gives me a comforting sense of security. It has no beginning and no end. It's very close and everywhere. I can live with that. I lapse into a kind of high, feeling free and without a care. Maybe that's what shock does to a person, but it all feels very easy. I'm walking through a different space and time. Singing. For hours.

Then a small light appears. And what if it's only the automatic lights of a small weather station? At the exact moment when I finally see the light I've been yearning for, I'm overcome with great doubt. I'm afraid the light won't deliver what I've been hoping for during the dark walk: help and relief. An end to this trial. What if no one is there to open the door? I hesitate, wanting to hang on my hope a little longer. *Okay, it's cold. Standing here is getting me nowhere. I have to get out of this situation as fast as possible.* I knock. Wait. After a few moments that seem endless to me I hear steps inside the little shack, and finally the promising sound of the lock turning. Very slowly the door opens, just a small crack. A young, sleepy face peeks carefully and distrusting through the slit. Questions are written on his face. But before he can put them into words, I answer them for him. "I had a car accident. On Gorge Trail. My truck is totalled. I saw your light on the way into the valley. Need your help."

They are students from the University of Sherbrooke in Quebec. They make me hot tea but otherwise seem to be helpless. Later, they tell me that they were scared when they heard my knock. And while one of them opened the door, someone stood behind him holding a kitchen knife. Just in case. They're acutely aware of how isolated their research station is. I ask them if they could drive me to the next telephone booth. It's a good thing my colleague Renee pushed so hard for a telephone line in our trailer at Highwood. She might see that differently right now, because I wake her from a deep sleep.

An hour later she picks me up at a lonely telephone booth in a parking lot in the valley. After a few hours of deep sleep, I start making phone calls. I call Carolyn Callaghan, for whom I work. She's also the owner of the truck, or what's left of it. Carolyn immediately sets off for the scene of the accident. In the meantime, I organize a towing service. And I contact the emergency service of the provincial park by radio. I want to know why I didn't reach anyone last night. The terse reply: "We only have someone on duty until 6:00 pm." Well then, I'll be sure to plan my next emergency during the agency's business hours.

We all plan to meet at the damaged truck. Renee and I are the first to arrive. Then we hear the tow truck approaching, squealing and sliding. Its tires spin; it won't make it to the truck. The driver has to turn around and exchange his truck for another vehicle with chains. It's icy, as smooth as glass. Renee stands there with her mouth hanging open, speechless, and that rarely happens. I stand next to her, appalled, staring at the truck lying upside down. Now, in full daylight, it looks really grotesque. I cannot believe I was sitting inside there and got away with nothing more than a case of shock and a scrape on my left pinkie finger that isn't even worth mentioning. It's clear that something protected me, something wanted me to go on living. I think about my sensing of my papa last night, and the inner peace and determination that filled me as I walked. Wolf Spirit, thank you for your perseverance!

WOLF SPIRIT 4
OCTOBER 2005

My room is at the very top, on the 11th floor, the neurological ward. One time, my friends manage to smuggle Nahanni into my room while someone distracts the nurses. Cheers for that! Outside my window, I can make out the silhouette of the Rocky Mountains far to the west. That gives a little familiarity to my new place here in a hospital bed. In the coming days, they'll do all kinds of tests in preparation for brain surgery. Phil sets up his work laptop next to my bed. He is almost always with me. Everything is moving so fast. That's a good thing. It's too fast for the news to sink into my consciousness – it came from nowhere and I was utterly unprepared. Completely incomprehensible to me. Why now, of all times? I finally have a wonderful partner, love my Nahanni; I'm just getting back from the experience of a lifetime, spending an entire afternoon in a meadow with the wild coastal wolves, and I can still feel the gentle touch of the leading female. We've made a great film about protecting the wolves, and I finally feel I have "arrived." And now this diagnosis: brain tumour, size of a golf ball, stage III, aggressive – average life expectancy, one and a half years.

Wild Encounters

LIVINGSTONE

MORNING MIST
EARLY SUMMER 2004

Damp, thick morning mist rises slowly from the Livingstone River. The Livingstone Range is in the midst of the international Crown of the Continent ecosystem that encompasses the Rocky Mountains of Alberta, British Columbia and Montana. It comprises an important connection between the protected areas of the Waterton–Glacier International Peace Park (which straddles the Canada–USA border) to the south and the Kananaskis–Banff complex to the north. Lying along the eastern flank of the Rockies, this mountain range includes many different ecosystems, from the gentle and often grassy, open foothills parkland through the subalpine to the alpine zone; it contains a great variety of habitats and thus myriad species. Just east of it are the bordering ranchlands where I have done many night watches in the most varied forms.

I huddle on a folding camp chair, wrapped up in my big blue down jacket. With a warm woollen hat pulled down low on my face, I hold a metal Thermos coffee cup with both hands. The hot, fragrant steam does me good. Thoughtfully I sip at it and feel the comforting warmth inside my body. The nights are still very cool here at 1200 metres, although it's already June. No one forces me to take a plunge into the river every morning to wash myself, but I love this ceremony. Afterward, you warm up, your whole body tingles and you feel truly ready for the day. A second cup of coffee can't hurt, especially because nothing is stirring yet in Dave's tent.

Slowly the fog lifts to reveal a view of the grassy slope on the other bank of the river, a little at a time. I can just see my coyote family slipping into some of the young aspen growth scattered around the hill-like islands. They are my morning entertainment. Sometimes I can observe them for longer periods, but often it's only a brief glimpse. I always enjoy the sight of their agility and playfulness. They're so wonderfully carefree. Maybe they take a swim every morning too? In reality they have no reason to romp through life so joyfully; they are certainly the least respected and most persecuted mammals in North America. Because these predators can reproduce quickly and lose their shyness in a pack – even in the presence of people – they seem to be almost omnipresent. That explains why they are seen as vermin and treated as such. Even since I once observed an entire coyote family along the Athabasca River north of Jasper for several hours in a row, I know they are much more endearing than their reputation. They actually tend to be loners, but when they start a family group, the clown in them is brought to life, and they enjoy each other's company.

I once met a hunter out stalking elk. Since then, in the spring of each year, he has sent me his coyote quota: his goal is to kill a hundred animals every winter. And he reaches this number every year, too. This hunter is a retired schoolteacher. Not a simple, uneducated man. And he always tells me how much he admires these animals when he has the opportunity to observe them. And then he kills as many of them as possible. Just like the ranchers. They believe the coyotes kill their newborn calves. Which they will do, in exceptional situations when they are out in the pasture unprotected by their mothers or people. But the coyotes' main source of food is rodents, especially pocket gophers, the little gophers that build tunnel systems throughout the fields by the millions. Along with birds of prey, coyotes are their natural enemies. The predators regulate the population and thereby also reduce the number of burrows. The holes at the entrances to the burrows cause great damage in the cattle industry, when cows step into the holes and break their legs. Then comes exactly the same rancher who shot the coyotes before, and he starts shooting the gophers. Or sometimes it's the rancher's children who do that; shooting gophers is a popular pastime among young adolescents who will become the next generation of ranchers. They learn early on what the rancher believes should be shot out of existence, which animals cause damage. But they don't learn that useful things must remain. They don't learn all the ways wild animals are useful. And they also don't learn that their actions unleash a cascade of undesirable consequences.

The coyotes have disappeared completely from my view, and it's getting to be time to chase Nahanni over to Dave's tent. He should get up, and Nahanni leaves him no other choice when she wags her tail exuberantly against the side of his tent. This is another morning ritual I love! I hear Dave's sleepy grumbling inside the tent, and shortly he peels himself out of it, stretches, and makes a beeline for the coffee, which, prepared by a good fairy, is already waiting for him. Now the research team is complete, if not yet completely ready for duty.

While we enjoy an extensive breakfast together, we study the map of our 1200-square-kilometre research area. We are working for the Miistakis Institute. Associated with the University of Calgary, the institute focuses on research dealing with environmental issues in the unprotected regions of southwest Alberta. It consists of an interdisciplinary team of young scientists under the leadership of Professor Mike Quinn. I feel very comfortable in this group. Mike hired me in the spring straight from my research work on the prairies. It was one of the few perfect transitions I have experienced from a completed project to the next one. At first I was on my own, but it was clear from the start that I would need reinforcement. That came in the form of Dave. We knew each other in passing; our paths had crossed while monitoring wolves in Kootenay National Park. We get along very well with each other.

It's turning out to be a beautiful summer, maybe the nicest one I've experienced in Canada. I love this landscape, and my "home," our remote tent site directly at the drop off to the Livingstone River, which has embedded itself about 30 metres deep in the earth here. Asked where I live, I laughingly answer, "Highway 40, Forestry Trunk Road, kilometre 46." There are little kilometre posts along the dusty, gravel logging road, as there are on all forest roads, so that people can radio each other their locations or – even more important – learn over the radio where a truck is thundering toward you. Then you hopefully have enough time to get out of the way. So near "kilometre 46" for this summer, we've stretched a plastic tarp between two aspen trees and set up our kitchen underneath it. Dave has a strong practical streak. He is an experienced camper and knows how to put together living quarters without four walls or a lot of supplies. The only problem we never completely resolve is the issue of our leftover food. Kilometre 46 is in the middle of bear territory – both black bears and grizzlies. A visit from these furry creatures is thus inevitable. So we stuff everything edible in our cars each morning after breakfast, but our camp is still never entirely bear-safe. I think that maybe Nahanni's presence and scent is deterrent enough for the bears. Or the thundering of those trucks. At any rate, we don't have a single bear incident in our camp. During the day while we're at work is a different story: Dave and I are looking after 24 camera traps, which we systematically hang on trees along the paths wildlife use and the ATV trails that run parallel to them.

As beautiful as Livingstone is, it is a region under extreme pressure. Enormous logging operations not only destroy habitat but also leave behind logging roads in the deepest valleys that have remained pristine until now. Exploratory crews looking for deposits of natural gas and "seismic lines" cut perfectly straight clearings every which way through the landscape; the areas alongside these gouges are studied for the presence of natural gas in the wake of purposefully induced earthquakes. They are wide enough that an ATV can use them comfortably. And there are thousands of them here, especially in the summer months and on the weekends.

The four-wheeled ATV, built to go anywhere, is one of Albertans' favourite toys. They pull them on their own trailers behind their often monstrous motorhomes into the farthest reaches of

Livingstone. Often four of them for a family of four: mini-ATVs are a hit with the youngsters. They park right at the river, wherever there's space, unload, and then take off on a modern family outing into nature. The children wear helmets; they hear, see, and smell nothing but their loud motors, their handlebars and the stink of exhaust. Then they drive home again. That was their experience of nature. Every time I see a family outing like this roar past me, it makes me desperately sad. Their machines often have two-stroke engines, extremely loud and polluting. If this is what these children remember when they are adults and think about what they learned about nature growing up, then I am deeply worried about our environment. Because what have these children actually experienced of the natural world on their ATVs, racing through nature and yet so far removed from it? Not the sweet-warm scent of the subalpine coniferous forest where they spent their weekend, or the many bird calls that constantly relate what's happening at the moment, like a "Facebook of the forest": indignant, quiet, cheerful and annoyed, all in turn. And they won't be able to remember the wild animals either, because they will not have seen them; the animals will have withdrawn completely from the loud noise.

As adults, what will it mean to these children to preserve natural habitats? What will they think is worth protecting? And what will they miss if it is lost forever? Things they have never perceived with their own senses will always be distant and foreign to them. They will be indifferent to them.

Nature, on the other hand, will remember their visits all too clearly and for a long time to come. They leave behind scars that only heal after a long time, if at all: deep trenches eroded in meadows and on floodplains that are thousands of years old and on steep slopes only covered with a thin layer of topsoil, large areas of abrasions on roots, new paths – carved out by daddy with a chain saw. When they get home again, the children have learned from their parents how they can have their way with nature. Not how nature can be useful to them. Yes, it makes me sad to witness this already advanced level of alienation from nature, right here in Livingstone.

When I hike along the ATV trails, I feel like an alien without a motor, only my hiking boots, quiet and slow. That's how many of the ATV riders see me, too: they stop and are curious why I'm walking here. Ask if my ATV had a flat and whether or not I need any help. Every time I think to myself, *Hey, you're really nice people. How is it that you're so careless about nature? We're all one, connected to everything that exists.* But then I stop my train of thought and remind myself that we live in a "fun society" that prioritizes one's own fun above all else, without consequences, without responsibility, maybe even without any consideration. Fun is the contemporary translation of wrongly understood "freedom." We're allowed to do anything that's fun. And we need more and more of it, more and more intense experiences to get that thrill, take it to the extreme, even take the ultimate risk. At the same time, a large poster hangs prominently in the display window of a sporting goods shop in Canmore, not too far away. It shows a cool, stylish climber hanging with one hand on a vertical wall. Next to it the ambiguous advertising slogan: "I don't need friends." A sign of the times.

I arrive at the GPS point we picked out on the map back in camp according to an ingeniously random strategy we have devised. That's where I hang the first camera trap. Then I move into the forest perpendicular to the ATV trail until I come across a well-frequented game trail and install the second camera. The third is supposed to be put in place near another game trail that is at least 200 metres away from the main route. After two weeks I will take these down and install them again according to the same pattern in a different location. So much for the research method. Our line of questioning? We want to find out the extent to which motorized tourism affects the behaviour of the local wildlife. Are the animals disturbed by it? If so, to what extent? Do they withdraw? Leave the area? Lots of relevant questions that are especially important because there's no end to the ATV boom in sight; on the contrary, a sharp increase is anticipated.

The region just outside Calgary, a city with a million residents, is feeling this trend acutely. The ATV industry is worth billions of dollars and has a correspondingly powerful lobby. Only with hard facts and incorruptible data does anyone have even a small chance to at least regulate this development a little. With posted quiet zones, for example. The cameras are intended to provide us with this data. They take pictures of everything that moves past them, interrupting the camera's infrared beam: wildlife, riders, hunters and of course all motorized vehicles. And cows, cows, cows. At the same time, the devices save information about the exact time and weather conditions for each image.

Every evening, we sit before a vast quantity of data that still needs to be entered into the computer after a long day in the field. But downloading the pictures is always the highlight of each day. It's like Christmas and Easter combined. What will appear this time? Lots of empty frames, mistakenly triggered by branches moving in the wind or by raindrops. But also things that ran or drove through the frame too fast. We will never solve these mysteries. Nonetheless, there remain many thousands of pictures that let us in on life in the wild in this region. What we find is astonishing: every animal species you can think of that inhabits the Rockies, except the extremely rare mountain caribou, which barely survives as a mini-herd of five individuals farther north, near Jasper. Otherwise, every creature is represented: moose, elk, white- and black-tailed deer, mountain goat and the Rocky Mountain bighorn sheep are the hoofed animals; the full contingent of large predators, including black and grizzly bear, wolf, coyote, fox, cougar, lynx and bobcat; and the weasel, marten, badger and wolverine are the weasel-like animals. In addition there are wild rabbits, mountain hare, squirrels, chipmunks and myriad birds of every species. And many of them with very entertaining expressions when they're captured on camera.

Those expressions also make it clear, however, that these cameras do not go entirely unnoticed as the manufacturers promise. We also find a camera with a lovely hole in its lens; its last pictures show a black bear approaching. Another hangs crookedly from a tree on the bank of a gravel road; the battery cover complete with batteries is lying on the ground. Its last images are of a curious elk cow that suddenly veers off the gravel path and climbs straight toward the camera. Then you just see her muzzle. How she got the batteries out remains her little secret. The pictures taken at night are in black and white, and the infrared flash that is supposed to be invisible to wildlife seems to irritate many of them nonetheless. And it frustrates us when we can only vaguely recognize some body part but for the life of us can't identify it, and have to throw that particular image in the trash with a sigh. There it's in good company with the several thousand cows that often hang out directly in front of our cameras for hours, the arrogant creatures. They cost us lots of time, nerves and storage capacity by doing so. But out in the field, they also generated many a smile.

The images that remain are compared to other data: When and where were ATVs underway versus when did animal movement take place? Are there correlations between the two data sets? Is there evidence of cause-and-effect relationships, or of change in animals' behaviour, influenced by motorized activities? The entire following winter I sit in front of a huge chart and try to decipher answers.

Although the data gathering continues for two more summer and autumn seasons, we are not able to deliver clear, statistically relevant results. Instead, two of our cameras disappear without a trace. Our studies don't seem to meet with everyone's approval.

The problem is not so much the data. More to the point is that we can no longer find an area free of ATV activity that would be large enough to serve as a control area. Have we come too late? The answer will probably remain foggy for now. But the morning fog always lifts eventually. You just have to hang around long enough.

ENCOUNTERS
EARLY SUMMER 2004

For efficiency's sake, Dave and I divide our work every morning. During the day we're on our own but at least know approximately where the other one is. After Dave has an encounter with a grizzly bear, he is uneasy being alone, so we set out together for a few days after that. But with each hour you spend outdoors you gain more confidence and become more comfortable, and so we soon part ways during the daytime again. I'm actually never alone, because I always have Nahanni at my side. She is the most competent colleague I could ever dream of. She reveals to me the nature surrounding me and is in many ways my translator. She lets me know if a sound is worth following up on, and she points out important smells. She is the extension of my senses. And irreplaceable. Only during direct contact with wolves and when I have to take a plane do I leave Nahanni at home.

We are hiking along an ATV trail when suddenly a grizzly bear trots around a bend in the road. It takes my breath away, even though I know, of course, that such an encounter could happen at any time. In such situations, our primal fears probably come into play, an unconscious reservoir of human experiences. Dogs have a different access to them. And even if every brochure for tourists suggests something completely different in the case of an encounter with a bear, I let my Nahanni continue to run off the line. She is a dog that makes her decisions very independently, and I can rely on her to do the right thing. Now she races ahead, barking; the fur on her neck bristles and she jumps up and down stiffly and upright on all four paws in front of the bear. The bear stands still, looks baffled, turns around and gallops off in the direction it just came from. Nahanni disappears, glued to its heels. I hear some crashing in the brush, then she returns panting, but proud. I praise her. Still, we have to continue in the very direction in which the grizzly disappeared. So I employ my preferred method to avoid further encounters: I speak to the bear somewhere out there in the brush in a loud, clear and calm voice. I explain to it why we have to pass by it again and that we won't bother it. Nahanni stays on the leash for the next few minutes.

A few years earlier I had a very unsettling encounter with a black bear. And I don't ever want to experience anything like that again.

It is my first summer in the Canadian coastal rainforest. I'm out on my own, without Nahanni. It's raining hard and I've forged deep into the interior of the island. Like almost everywhere in this region, the undergrowth is very dense, which gives you only a very limited view. I hear a cracking, then he's already right in front of me: a large black bear – with his head down. That is not good. That position lets me know that he has already perceived me but didn't run away. I start to talk with him and tell him that I'm retreating. "I don't want to disturb you. Sorry if I've bothered you. I was already leaving anyway." The bear circles around me, then follows me. I get that creepy feeling that accompanies an immediate threat. I start to sing "Hey Jude" by the Beatles, over and over, never stopping. Over seven minutes in length, "Hey Jude" was the longest single of all time when it was released in 1968. As I sing, I experience some of the longest minutes of my life. The bear follows me, and he's no longer just curious, that's clear now. If he switches definitively into hunting mode, I'll have to react quickly. At regular intervals, I turn around: he's still there, and getting closer. I try to reach my project leader, Chris, on the radio. He responds.

"Chris, a black bear is after me. I'm on the left side of the river above the waterfall."

"Don't let the bear out of sight and cross the river immediately. I'm coming toward you on the game trail there." I can hear the concern in his voice.

The rain gets heavier and I can hardly see the bear, but I sing louder. Then I reach the river. I can cross it without difficulty. The bear remains standing on the shore, indecisive. I don't even want to know if he gets into the water. As soon as I'm on the game trail, I run down the path at full speed. I meet Chris near a big spruce. He gives me a hug that's short but long enough that I can tell how relieved he is. The bear isn't following me anymore. For a few moments we both stand there, leaning against the tree, simply standing there.

Bears are intelligent animals and develop personalities of incredibly varied character. I never assume that a bear is one of the animals that innately has it in for us humans. And why should it? Bears are omnivores, but more than 75 per cent of their diet is plants. The bears on the coast have a higher protein consumption, but the protein practically swims into their mouths three mouths out of the year: there's an abundance of salmon. During this period, the loners are quite sociable and tolerate several of their kind nearby. And people don't have to be too worried during this time, as long as they treat the bears with respect. Black bears, however, have a reputation of being more aggressive than grizzly bears.

In the past decade, a steady stream of bear tourism has developed in British Columbia. Visitors from around the world are enticed to so-called "bear-viewing lodges," from which they are brought to specially built platforms where they can observe the bears fishing, up close without either party being disturbed. Both the operators of these businesses and the environmental protectionists can be proud of the fact that in British Columbia this kind of bear marketing now brings in more tax revenue than destructive grizzly bear hunting. Not to mention the impressive experience of being able to observe these giants at close range in a peaceful and safe setting. Here, once again, the animals are their own best ambassadors for the potential of cohabitation. Dean Wyatt, owner of the Knight Inlet Lodge, one of the most renowned of such bear lodges, had this to say about it in a report issued by the Raincoast Conservation Foundation: "My guests shoot the bears at least 20,000 times a year, but always with a camera." In 2007 alone, Wyatt earned a profit of more than C$3.1-million with his enterprise. His property is home to about 30 bears, so the value of a bear can be estimated at approximately $100,000. By comparison, hunters, hunting guides and their guests are allowed to shoot and kill up to 320 grizzly bears in British Columbia each year with the permission of the authorities. This hunting brings in 3.3 million Canadian dollars, or $10,300 per bear, which is one-tenth the value of an ecological bear-viewing economy. Those are only rough estimations of course, but they point clearly to the truth behind the figures: a live bear is worth much more than a dead one. And not only in purely economic terms.

The bear's value for the ecological system, and especially the emotional impact of the experience that all people who have ever been so close to a great bear carry with them for the rest of their lives, which are much harder to evaluate, are not even part of that equation. In light of such facts, I don't understand why grizzly bear hunting is still tolerated at all. Typically the animals are baited or lured to a certain spot, then shot from a raised blind. Anyone who feels proud and brave doing that can only be pitied.

Ian McAllister is one of the foremost grizzly bear experts. His anecdotes about encounters with the "great bear," as grizzlies are also called, are convincing because they are genuine. And the First Nations Elders living along the coast relate that earlier, the women, often quite slender, would go into the forest when the berries were ripe and gather the fruits side by side with the great brown beasts. If they got too close to each other, the women would talk to the bears in their traditional language. And the bears recognized that these people presented no danger to them. McAllister has discovered something similar. According to his theory, grizzlies react more aggressively from the start when they come across a hunter or someone with a gun. It's possible that their excellent sense of smell perceives the metal or other parts of the weapon that send clear, threatening signals to them. Or, conscious of their weapon, armed people signal their dominance and dangerousness to the bear, possibly even subconsciously through their body language. Or the bear simply *senses* the overly confident attitude of people carrying guns.

Since 1995, when Italian neurophysiologist Dr. Giacomo Rizzolatti and his team officially presented their discovery – based on research with primates – of what are called mirror neurons, we finally have proof that non-verbal communication is very real and can trigger reproducible reactions or even emotions in the brains of others. Although research has not yet been done with other species, it makes sense to me that this ability is not limited to primates but also exists in many other highly developed mammals. Especially those that live in highly social groups, such as wolves, and those that can be dangerous for each other, like bears. It will definitely be interesting to see what more will be discovered in this field of research in coming years. For me it's clear that the familiar expression "what goes around, comes around" conveys an old wisdom that we shouldn't ignore, especially when it comes to sensitive wild animals with their finely tuned "antennae." The First Nations in North America, like all Indigenous peoples, have embedded this wisdom in their legends, religions and everyday life.

One time, for example, Lone Wolf, of the Heiltsuk First Nation, is standing in the middle of wolf territory in his neon-orange rain gear. He is wearing the exact opposite of a camouflage outfit, the opposite of what we would consider appropriate. When Chris carefully brings it up with him, Lone Wolf quickly has a convincing answer for him: "Nobody wanna be sneaked on." In other words, no one appreciates being stalked unawares. He finds that it is much more honest and constructive to openly show yourself to the animals. Lone Wolf simply imagined himself in the animals' position and then transferred his own feelings to them: his honesty and a kind of casualness toward them. Have the animals perhaps felt these emotions stirring in themselves?

During my very close encounters with wolves I, too, often had the impression that they could sense my emotions. Or even more: that they want to pass something on to me that will help me with the great challenge that lies ahead.

WOLF SPIRIT 5
OCTOBER 2005

Foothills Hospital, Tom Baker Cancer Centre, Calgary. First patient briefing about the therapy ahead in a small, spare room without a window. Mutti, Phil, Mike and I are waiting for Dr. Easaw, my oncologist, and Dr. Sung, my radiologist for the coming months. A short, delicate and brutally realistic Asian woman enters the room and introduces herself. "How much do you want to know?"

"Everything."

Then she tells me the precise diagnosis, the planned therapy and the survival rate. Clear, factual, shattering. And finally the sentence: "But hope dies last." And she's done. But hope dies last. Yes, that's exactly right, doctor. *That's* what I'll remember! I don't want to be a statistic, I'm embracing hope! And suddenly it seems like I feel a starter's gun go off deep inside me. The race of my life has begun. The race FOR my life.

Wolf Spirit, hold on! Because hope dies last.

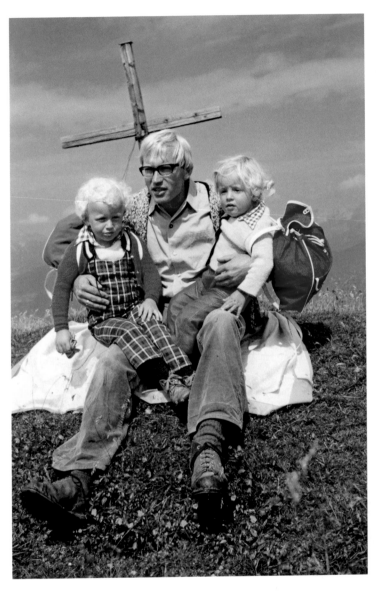

From an early age, my sister Gerhild (left) and I (right) gathered mountain peaks with our papa like other girls collected dolls.

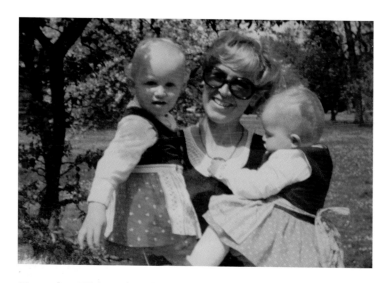

My mother, Edeltraud, with my sister and me at a park in Radstadt, 1973

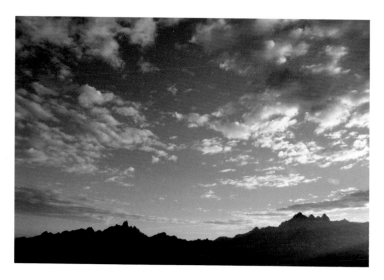

The Gosaukamm in the Austrian Alps, at sunrise

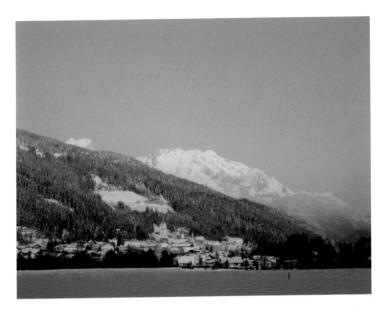

My home town, Radstadt, Austria

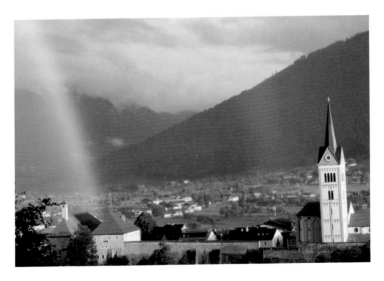

Radstadt at the foot of a rainbow

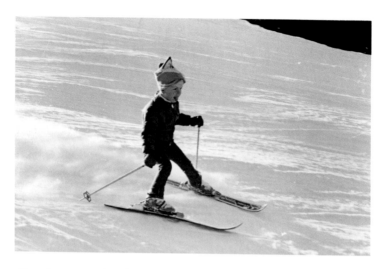

Already very much at home in the snow at the age of four

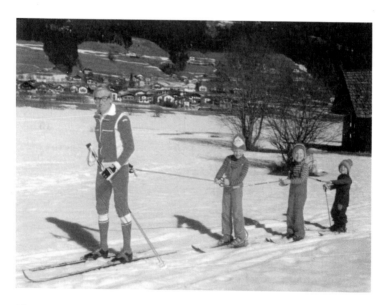

The wintertime Pflüger train at home in Radstadt, Austria

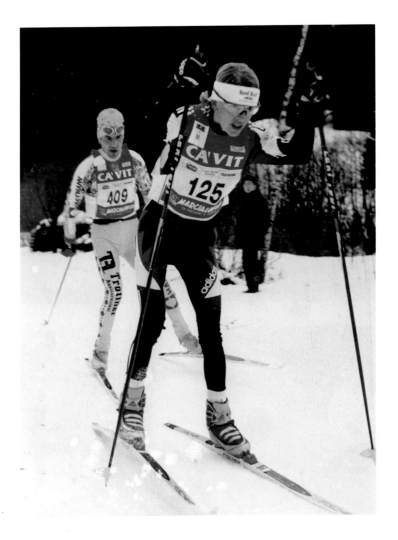

24° Marcialonga di fiemme e fassa   26 gennaio 1997

Taking part in one of the biggest and fastest cross-country races in the world, the Marcialonga, in Italy, 1996

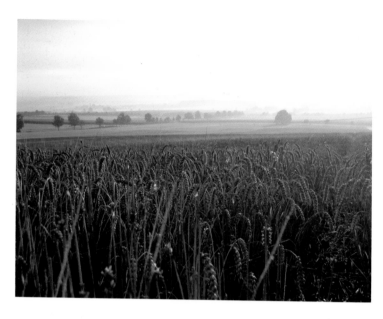

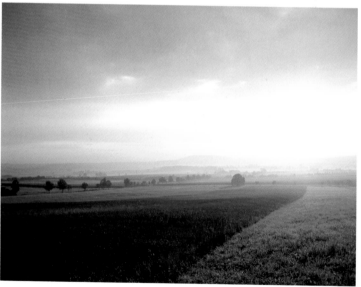

Autumn field just before the harvest in Markt Berolzheim, Germany

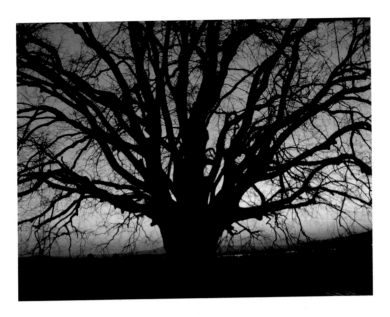

Power tree in Markt Berolzheim, Germany

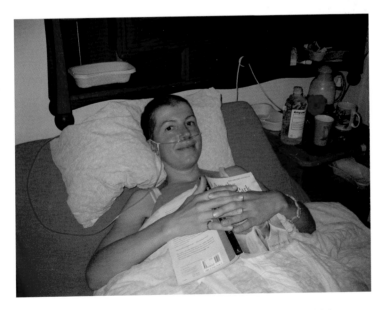

Viral therapy at Dr. Thaller's clinic in Bavaria, Germany, 2006

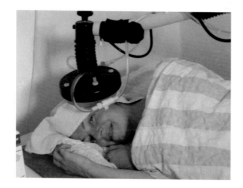

*Hyperthermia treatment
at Dr. Thaller's clinic*

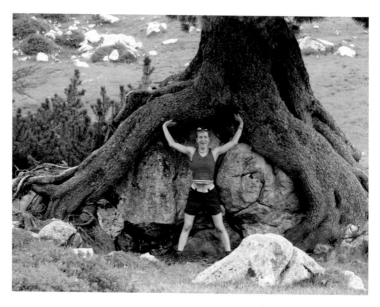

Getting stronger again!

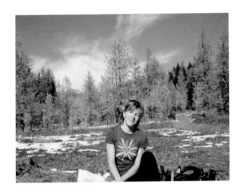

Fall colours at Healy Pass, Banff National Park

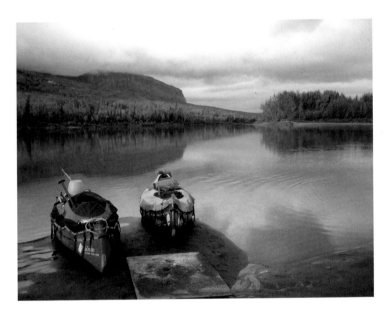

The end of a great journey on the Nahanni River, Northwest Territories, shared with great friends

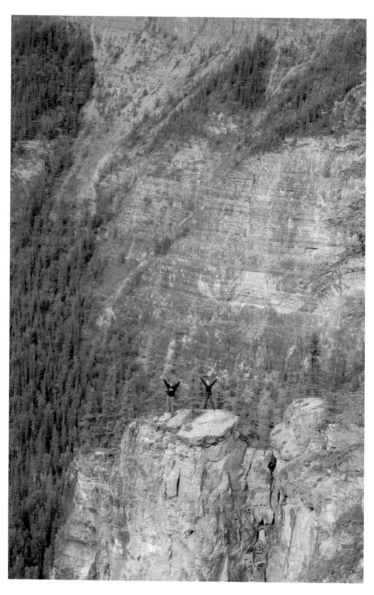

Triumphant atop the Gate, a feature of the Nahanni River,
Northwest Territories

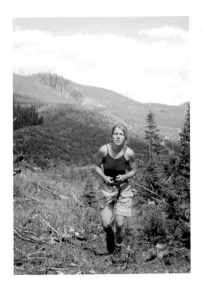

Crossing clearcuts while checking wildlife cameras in southwestern Alberta.

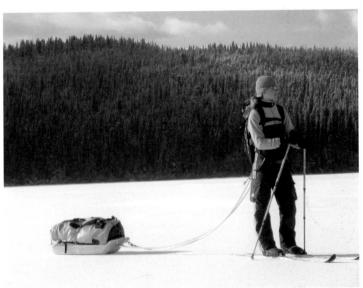

On the trail of the wolves with a wildly unstable children's bobsled in Canada, 2003

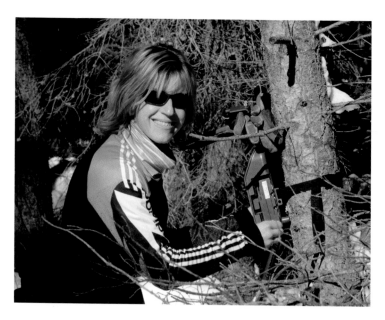

Tending to one of the infrared cameras set up to capture images of wildlife

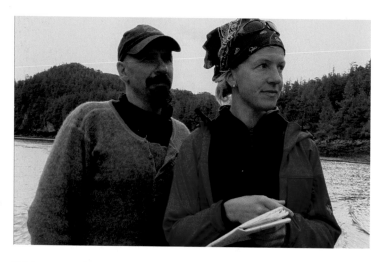

With captain Jean Marc, approaching a remote island off the coast of BC in search of coastal wolves

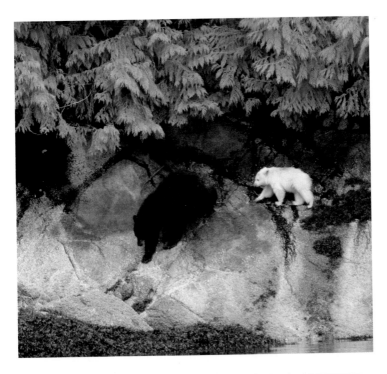

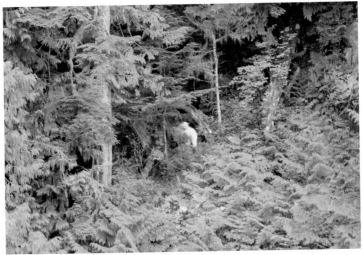

Great Bear Rainforest, BC

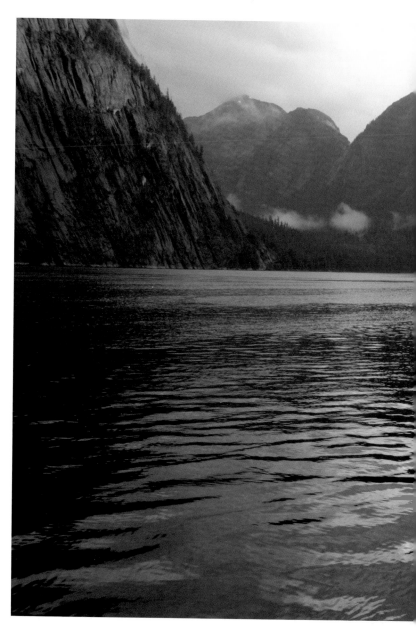

Evening settles on board the research boat "Achiever," Great Bear Rainforest

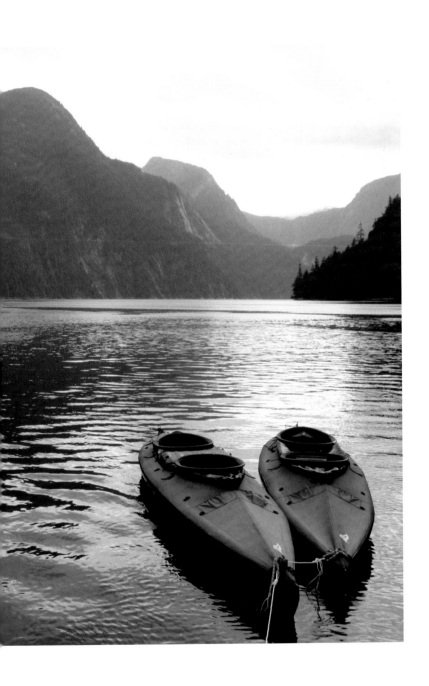

An early morning boat ride in the Great Bear Rainforest, BC

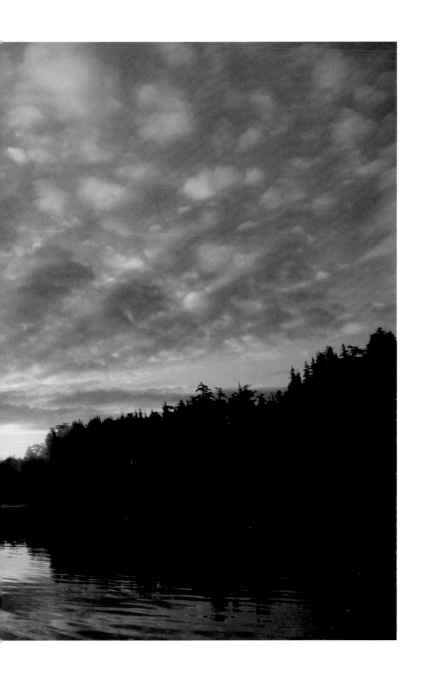

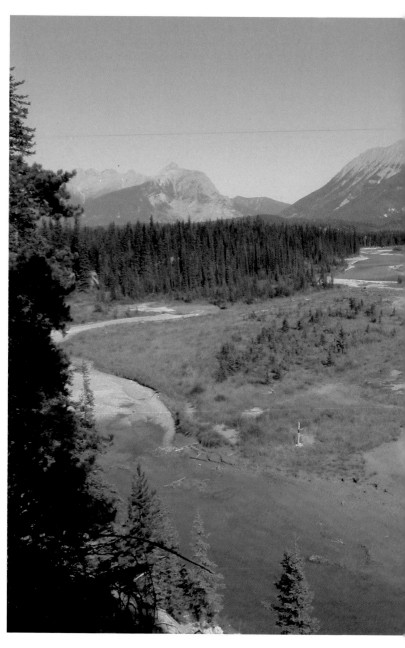

Outlook from the Dolly Varden Trail along the Kootenay River

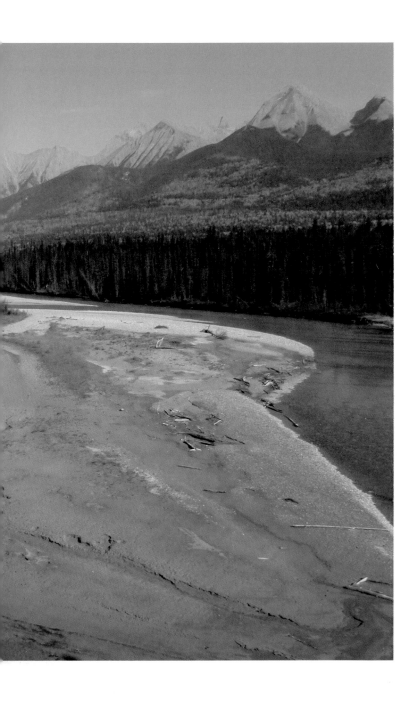

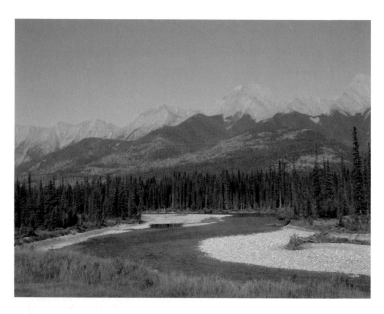

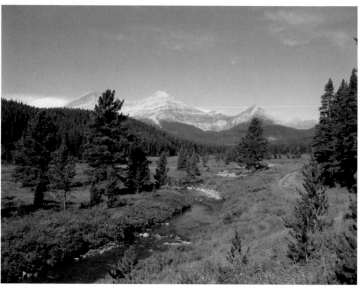

top: *Kootenay River in Kootenay National Park, BC*
bottom: *The upper course of the Oldman River against the Rocky Mountains – my "office" in the Livingstone Range in Alberta, 2004*

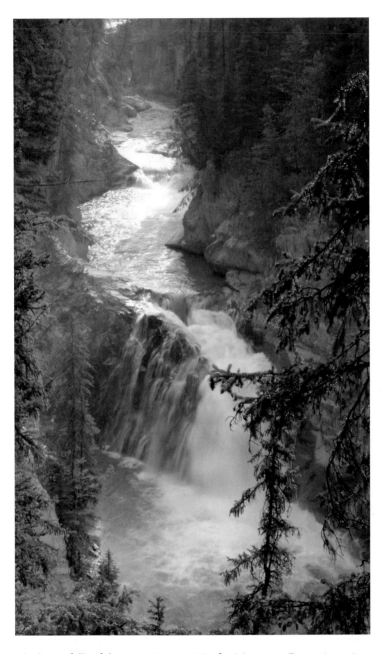

The lower falls of the Cross River at Nipika Mountain Resort in spring

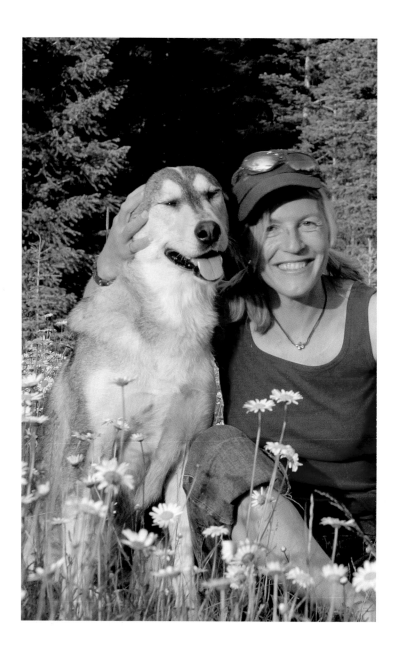

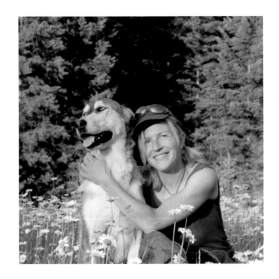

*Content and
happy with my
Nahanni in a
sea of daisies at
Nipika*

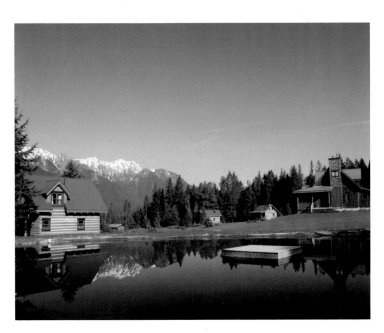

Nipika, my home in Canada

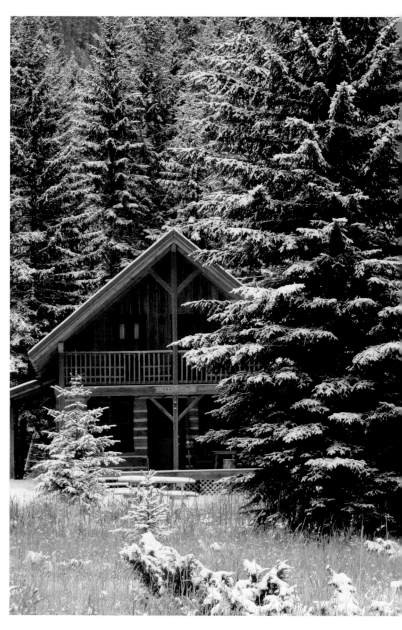

Visitors at Nipika

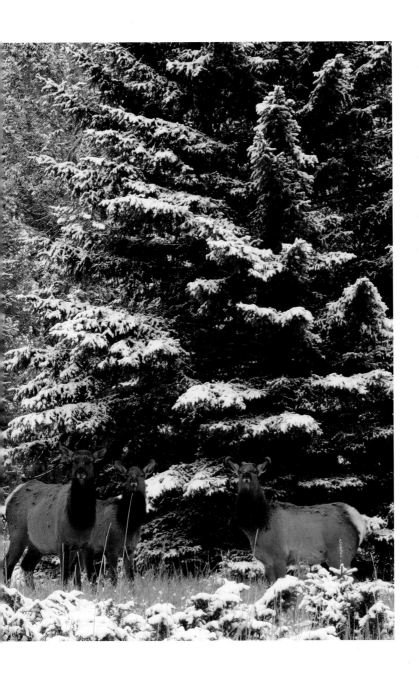

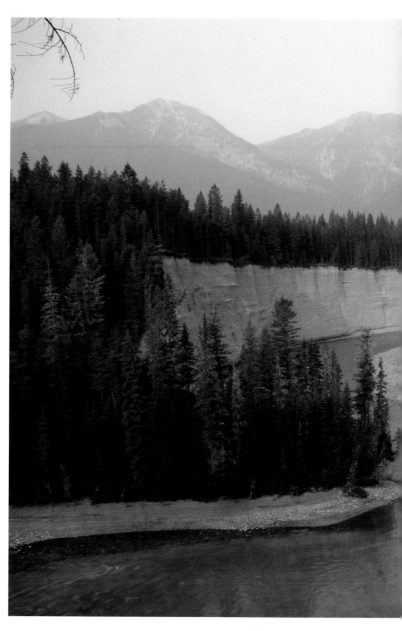

A bend in the Kootenay River at Nipika Beach

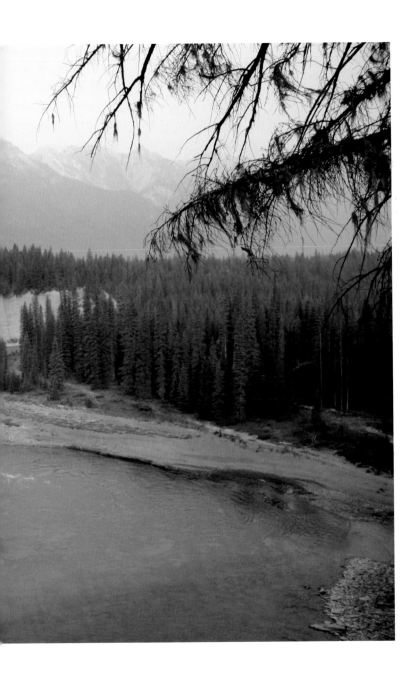

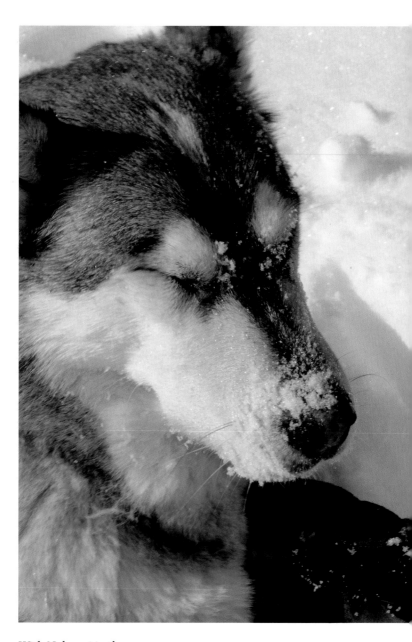

With Nahanni in the snow

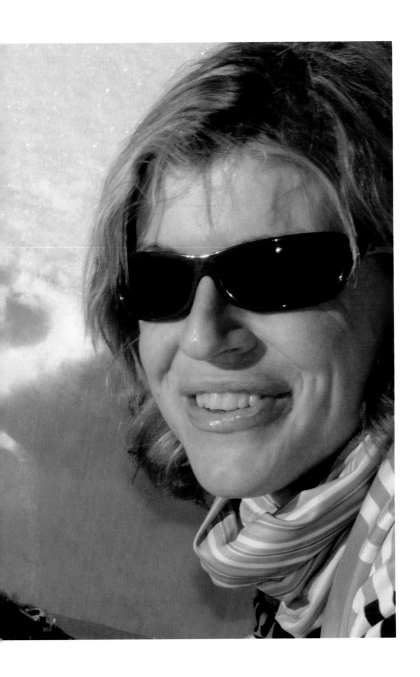

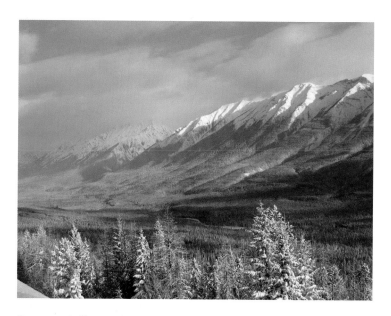

Kootenay Valley, my winter workplace

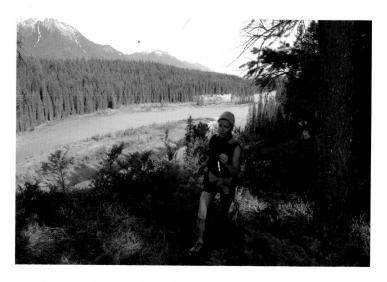

Running part of the Nipika trail system along the Kootenay River

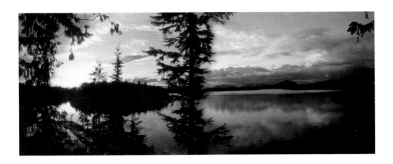

View from the cabin during Chris's and my stay at Ian and Karen McAllister's place in the Great Bear Rainforest, my most favourite place on the Kootenay River

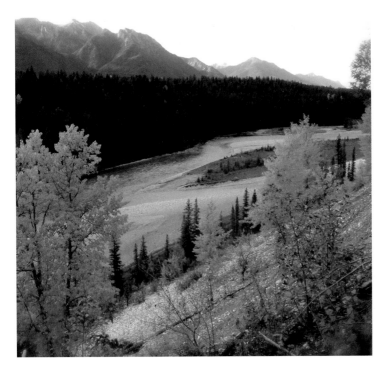

The Kootenay River at Nipika Mountain Resort

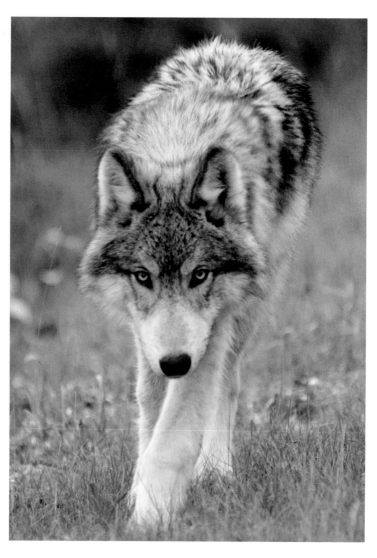

The wolf, the soul of the forests

Every Step Counts

ADVENTURES IN THE WORLD OF SPORTS

HOLD ON
WINTER 1997

As long as we have hope, we are alive. Or in other words, never give up! Always believe you'll reach your destination! One of the greatest lessons I took away from elite endurance sports was exactly that: the race is only over when you've crossed the finish line. During a 50-kilometre, 70-kilometre or even 90-kilometre ski race, at every metre you have the option to simply not take the next step and to get off the course. Not wanting to continue subjecting yourself to this, this exertion to the point of pain, at the same time knowing that the situation won't end so soon – in fact it's likely to get worse – and that with every step you're getting closer to exhaustion but also to the goal. For a large part of the race, the body dictates the motions, especially at the beginning; but the longer it lasts, the more your physical strength ebbs. But we are also mind and will power. And those facets can take the lead, dramatically jumping in when the body can't go any farther. That's when the liminal experience begins, a condition in which you look something larger straight in the eyes.

In the course of my athletic career, my will often urged my body beyond my normal limits, and pushed them back a little farther each time. Someone once said to me, "Watch out, once you've given up in the middle of a race, you'll do it again and again. You get used to doing the easy thing." So giving up became "not an option" for me. One time, I paid the price for it, during the Norwegian Birkebeinerrennet, a long-distance cross-country ski race. Up to that point, I was ranked third in the overall standings of the Worldloppet, the world cup of marathon cross-country ski racing, and had the chance to move further up the ladder. So I flew to Oslo and from there drove to Rena, a small village in the middle of nowhere on the side of the mountain that is to be conquered during the race. On the other side of it is Lillehammer, site of the 1994 Winter Olympics, and the goal. Between them lie an endless ascent, a broad and lonely plateau and then a long descent into Lillehammer. I never reached the descent because I stepped off the track in the middle of the plateau at the Red Cross station at kilometre mark 30 (out of a total of 54 kilometres). More was not possible with the fever I already had when I arrived. What I didn't know was that it was a two-hour car ride to Lillehammer. I was put on a 50-seat bus – by now terribly feverish – and told, "When the bus is full, we'll all drive to Lillehammer together." The bus stayed empty. Hours went by and the skiers who threw in the towel at precisely this checkpoint remained few. In the meantime, at a small wooden hut not far from the bus, I was introduced to the Norwegian method of fighting fever: litres and litres of the strongest black coffee. A small transistor radio provided boisterous live commentary on the race in the background. In Norwegian, of course. The only thought in my head was that I had to be in Lillehammer for the awards ceremony – the awards ceremony for the entire Worldloppet would also take place there, and in spite of everything, I could still end up in third place.

For the descendants of the Vikings, however, that was no reason to start the bus's engine any sooner to drive me to Lillehammer on time. "You can always take a taxi," was the bus driver's emotionless suggestion. A two-hour taxi ride in Norway? That would have cost me more than the modest prize money that third place would pay out. When we finally arrived in Lillehammer, it was all over. And when I just caught the president of the Worldloppet organization by his coattails, he handed me a cheque for the prize money, minus 25 per cent, because I hadn't been physically present at the awards ceremony.

Even the legend of the Norwegian Birkebeinerloppet, so rich in tradition, relates the importance of never giving up and continuing to hope to the very end. Without this attitude, the Birkebeiner – the king's warriors, who protected their shins from the deep and often cutting snow with the bark of the birch tree – probably wouldn't have reached their goal. In the year 1205 a civil war was raging in Norway. To protect the young Prince Haakon from the rival challengers, the "Baglers," the Birkebeiner took the little boy to a safe place on the other side of the mountain. Even today, all participants in the Birkebeiner race have to wear a backpack weighing 3.5 kilograms, the weight of the king's young son.

The great lessons related to not giving up play a huge part in my story too. The Transjurassienne in 1997, the French Worldloppet race, 72 kilometres. Rain falls in the morning, later wet snow, the conditions are brutally slow, and my legs have already withstood a lot of long races this season. The course is a big loop. Several times Papa stands at the side of the road and coaches Boti, Mikhail Botvinov and me. At the halfway point, I can hardly put one foot in front of the other, and my inner demons are howling and screaming the question: *Why are you torturing yourself like this? Why are you doing this to yourself? STOP IT!* And the worst part is, I have no reasonable answer, no convincing argument to keep going. Just one: because I'm already doing it. It's a kind of delirium. And that is alarming, because I know how fast "it doesn't matter" creeps in, the most dangerous of all feelings, numbing and will-zapping. *No, go away, get lost!* One step, it would just be one step, not forward, but to the side, off the track and out of the race and the pain. I stay in the race. And slowly I notice that my fellow competitors are in the same boat as me; some of them are in even worse shape. I start to overtake other skiers, first one, then another one, then more and more. And at some point I cross the finish line, in second place. The points I earn are important to the overall world-cup rankings. I've never been so close to quitting, and I don't believe I've ever come so close to my absolute limits. And still I make it to the finish line, and am the second one across. At the time, I couldn't begin to imagine the immense significance this experience would have for me eight years later.

WOLF SPIRIT 6
OCTOBER 2005

I want to get healthy again. I promise myself not to give up, to hang in there. Endurance is something I have learned, not least from wolves. They are the endurance athletes of the animal kingdom. Moving at an average speed of 8 kilometres per hour, they can cover distances up to 100 kilometres per day. They roam 1500 kilometres and more from their home territory. In the process, they master seemingly insurmountable obstacles or barriers, repeatedly and without being noticed. The farther the female wolf moves away from her family group, the greater the danger for her that she'll never be able to return; in new territory there are many dangers she isn't familiar with and that she hasn't experienced in the protective circle of the pack or learned about from her parents. But she presses on. Endurance is one of the most legendary characteristics of wolves. And to have endurance is also to have the ability to devote yourself to something unconditionally. To tenaciously pursue a goal, patiently making your way and confidently moving forward. The most important thing, and the hardest, is that endurance takes time. Time that isn't measured by the minute and second hands of a clock but by the development of your own character. Endurance is character-building. At the start is inexperience, immaturity. It defines the desire to arrive at some point. In between is the learning, the maturing. The actual path.

When I follow the traces of wolves for hours, their focused tracks tell me about their endurance and their search for prey, usually far too distant to see, and for success beyond the horizon. It's true that it is impossible to definitively distinguish between a wolf and a dog on the basis of a single paw print. But if you follow the trail for a while, the linear pattern of the individual tracks soon verifies that it's a wolf in a sustained trot: it moves efficiently through the terrain and hardly lets itself be distracted from its route.

During the interview for my first job in wolf research, I quickly noticed that endurance is also a very important attribute of a good field biologist: psychic as well as physical endurance. I always got good results in the latter in sports medicine examinations. I have an exceptionally high vo_2 max, or maximal oxygen uptake rate. That means my lungs can take in a very high proportion of oxygen, the precondition for good endurance performance. Even if these sports performance exams are always a horror for me, they do provide some useful data points. Otherwise, I minimize technical controls. I believe in the wisdom in my body, and over the years I've learned to both understand it and to torture it.

Of course, at the beginning, I also trained with a heart-rate monitor strapped to my chest and wore the corresponding pulse monitor on my wrist. But the monitor leads to far too much dependence on technology. Many people rely on the digital readout on their wrist like drivers looking to their dashboard to know how fast they're driving. But we are not machines; we are people and cannot be reduced to a number. We are feeling creatures. But we can also learn and forget. That's why I train not only my body but also my perception of various intensities. I learn to assess myself. And I can't think back to a single race in which I had to seriously reduce my level of performance toward the end. Endurance also means being fully present with all your energy to the very end.

Like the wolf, which follows its prey with enormous endurance and after hours or even days still has power for the last spurt, a successful hunt. I take the wolf as my role model. I don't give up.

THE EDGE OF THE FOREST
WINTER 1981–1986

Finally we are moving into our new house. It is a log house and smells wonderfully like the forest. The big trees right behind it are thickly covered with snow. My parents worked all summer long on the construction alongside friends, acquaintances and the new neighbours. Now it stands there, unfinished, but is declared good enough to be a new home for our family of five. Besides, tomorrow is Christmas. The new house will be the best gift ever. It's snowing hard and the steep driveway to the little development above the roofs of Radstadt will be a great challenge for anything on four wheels. The Kaswurm family's tractor helps haul the few pieces of furniture from our rental apartment down in the valley up to the new, lofty heights on the slopes of the Rossbrand, a nearby mountain peak. It's all so exciting for us three children. My sister Gerhild and I are just 13 months apart; Gerhild is ten, I'm nine, and my brother Volker is six.

We've already romped around on the construction site all summer long and were more of a hindrance than a help, that's for sure, especially for our mother. At one point Volli, as Volker is called, broke through the makeshift roof boards and plunged to the ground. Once again, his guardian angel intervened. As so often.

But most of the time we would rather be out in the woods, anyway. The forest begins on my parents' property, right behind the new house, and we all find that more interesting than anything else. From then on we live at the edge of the forest. And the neighbourhood kids are all about our age: at least nine new playmates with plenty of creative ideas and the urge to explore. The afternoons, especially, we spend in the woods. Indians chase cowboys chase Indians chase cowboys chase robbers chase police chase robbers. One time, the cowboys tie me to a tree (= stake; I always want to be one of the Indians) so tightly that I had bruises for a long while. The horse game is great too. Some of us are horses, the rest are the riders who attach the "horses" to long ropes – sorry, of course I mean *reins* – and direct them through the woods. Or the dog game, just like with the horses except the "dogs" bark instead of neighing and have to lift a leg. Later we bravely face off against our "enemies" from other areas of the town in mud battles and search for their secret hiding places in the forest.

During our middle years in school, our time in the woods becomes a little more systematic. We become limnologists who precisely measure the water level in the little brook every day. In addition we are cacti collectors, tadpole breeders, turtle owners and transect inspectors. This last one we call "walking through the forest barefoot along a straight line." It's the crowning event of all our activities, only for the really hardened of us. The "little ones" – Volli, for example – aren't allowed to take part, of course, under any circumstances. Where the smaller children prove themselves valuable is in the nearly annual circus and theatre performances in the neighbour's garden. Volli's masterful appearance as a cuckoo on the roof of the garden shed remains legendary.

Of course, we are also children of our times: we often play with Playmobil – but we frequently take the boxes into the forest and build our forts and castles and whatever else is important there. In bad weather I can't get enough of the series of books about Tina and Tini, two friends who put an end to all kinds of criminal activities. And the *Five Friends*. And I have my horse books; I know all the breeds by heart, as befits a girl of that age and a future horse owner. From my perspective there are no financial disadvantages to horse ownership, since I'll never need to buy a car. I can just take my horse everywhere I want to go. My parents think in somewhat smaller terms: the turtle Elena joins our family. She belongs out in the yard, too. Papa bores a hole through the end of her shell and we attach a long string to it so she can roam the yard almost freely all summer long – just like us.

Once a week I have a standing appointment inside our four walls: when a new episode of the television series *Grizzly Adams* is on. Otherwise, the TV isn't turned on very often. Its time is in the winter, when the whole family eagerly watches just about every ski race that's broadcast live. Papa is president of the ski club in a place that hardly has its equal in the number of elite winter athletes it has produced and continues to produce, in every skiing discipline: star athletes in alpine, cross-country, ski jumping, biathlon and Nordic combination.

Radstadt itself lies embedded between the Northern Limestone Alps (*Kalkalpen*) and the Alpine divide to the south, in what is called the Grauwacken zone, or Grasberg region. And it's a snow hole. The entire region thrives on winter tourism. To ensure that it remains internationally prominent, youngsters from the area are strongly supported in their sport disciplines. Every toddler learns to ski here, of course. Mutti frequently takes us out on the slopes. At the T-bar lift, the scene is thus: Gerhild slipping and sliding next to Mutti, with me between her legs and Volli hanging firmly tucked under her arm. According to family legend, a German man on holiday once asks her if she does this professionally – he has two more toddlers for her. But for unknown reasons, the three of her own are enough. Mutti never tires of showing us our homeland from above, even when we are very young. We collect mountain peaks like others collect stamps. She got that from her father. After working all week, every weekend he would ride into a valley by train and bike to climb up into the mountains. From there he always let loose his cheerful cry of joy, which we children hear from him live back down in the valley before a plate of schnitzel.

Mutti is also a trained pharmacist, which in her day still meant recognizing everything that is green and has healing properties, even when it's dried and crumbled. That too had an impact on us. Volli at least was able to get out of the "thrilling" botany lessons without a fuss.

In the winter we ski. At first downhill, of course, but at the age of 12 I switch to cross-country for good. We are a tight-knit little group, skiing in the forest and taking tours through the mountains. The training methods and the atmosphere suit me well. Our trainer, Hannes, knows not only how to get young teenagers racing through the woods but especially how to motivate them. So we have a little team mascot, for example, that we bring to every race and which the whole team throws into the air when one of us makes it to the podium. There's a team song to go with it, too: *"Aber bitte mit Sahne!"* ("With Whipped Cream, Please!") In the winter of 1985, Hannes packs the whole troop into the ski club minibus for a trip to the Nordic World Ski Championships in Seefeld, in Tirol. Amazing! There's even a chance we might get to see the great athletes Gunde Svan and Grete Ingeborg Nykkelmo up close and personal! The father of Dagmar and Bianca, two of my teammates, works for a big ski company in the next town over. He actually does arrange a meeting with Grete Ingeborg Nykkelmo, the star Norwegian skier. And we are given a signed autograph card. During the ride home I start to dream of driving to another world championship, not as a spectator this time but as a participant, a very successful competitor, the best one of all!

In the coming winter seasons, I consistently work my way up from district and regional competitions to the Austria Cup and the Austrian championships. At 13 I convince my parents to let me attend the Schigymnasium Stams, a boarding school in the province of Tirol that trains promising skiers. Papa is in favour, in his very understated but very supportive way. He himself was a track and field athlete while he was a student. And so he lets us kids do everything that was made possible for him. Mutti is less enthusiastic. She comes from a family in which she couldn't pursue the profession she wanted due to their financial situation. Nonetheless, I go to Stams. The entrance exam takes place in April 1986, just a few days after the atomic catastrophe at Chernobyl. We're out on a glacier in the most glorious weather, right where no one ought to be at the time, actually. But such a short time after the first official level 7 event on the International Nuclear Event Scale, no one really knows what it means and how people should react. It doesn't occur to us to suddenly change our plans and risk our dreams just because of an incident far away to the east.

Twenty years later, I think back on those hours in which I was exposed to an enormously high level of radiation. When I asked my oncologist in Canada if he has an explanation as to why I, of all people, got a brain tumour, he replied, "Destiny." Fate. I never ask that million-dollar question again. It's clear that there is no humanly comprehensible answer.

Following the entrance exam, I am accepted on probation, only due to my ability to jump. In terms of conditioning, I'll need to catch up to my colleagues, who already train very regularly. And I have my first bout of anemia, a condition that regularly accompanies me, and limits me, during my time in elite athletics.

Sometimes it's so bad that pills aren't enough to fill up the stores of iron in my body. I need injections of an aggressive iron compound. The first times I receive them they cause a systemic shock; I'm suddenly very hot and can hardly breathe. The liquid stings inside my veins and burns a little more each time. But you get used to lots of things. Especially when you have ambitious goals. I fully understand that I'm in Stams now, the number one crucible for Austrian skiers. Although I am only 14, I see this privilege as an entree to professional sports. And I know that I have to prove myself. Otherwise I won't return next year.

It is the first time that I train extensively, and it pays off in the wintertime with the first important successes. I want more, and therefore I need to weigh less. Three of us six girls start to pay attention to our weight. Our Czech trainer, Josef, encourages us to do so. This is the time when the two cross-country skiing styles that are commonplace today, classical and skate skiing, part ways once and for all. Especially in the realm of skate skiing – skiing with gliding steps, pushing side to side in a skating motion – with the technology and information available at the time, the lighter skiers have an advantage. It's more of a hovering dance on the snow; the trails are nothing more than wide, firmly packed paths of snow, while in classic cross-country, your skis glide in two parallel grooves. From the first, I love the freedom of skating. The lightness of the movement, gliding over the glistening snow. A new star rises in the international cross-country firmament as well: the years of Stefania Belmondo begin. The little Italian weighs barely 45 kilograms and flies from victory to victory with unbelievably quick strides. She also ushers in an era of the new, feminine cross-country skiers, replacing the "Eastern Bloc powerhouse" stereotype.

By nature I have a strong build, and my muscles respond quickly to progressive training. But I want to look like the new ideal and soon realize that the combination of training a lot and eating little can help me realize my goal. So that's just what I do. And then it doesn't matter who interjects – coach, parents, fellow athletes – I stick with it. I want to prove to everyone that I know best what the optimal way is. I have everything perfectly under control. But gradually a delusion begins to control me. The need to be more perfect than perfect, lighter than light. In spring I become thin, too thin. At the end of the first year of school and after a successful winter season, Papa and Mutti pick me up in Stams and bring me back to the forest's edge.

NO MAN'S LAND
SUMMER 1991

In Radstadt I try all summer long to gain enough strength to be able to return to Stams. But in vain. I will finish high school and get my Matura in Radstadt. On the afternoons when we don't have classes, I work out systematically and all by myself. Because my energy and strength are limited, I carefully consider which techniques and training methods are most efficient. More than anything, I develop a paradox, a finely tuned awareness of my body, which I then ignore. During these three years, I don't participate in a single competition, no sports-medicine testing or diagnostic performance evaluations. After I finish high school, I'd like to study forestry or landscape architecture or something like that. I'm interested in several degrees offered at BOKU, the University of Natural Resources and Life Sciences, in Vienna. And therein lies the problem for me. It's a major city and far away from snow. But I absolutely want to become a top cross-country skier, and in my opinion that's impossible to reconcile with attending university in Vienna. My strategic alternative is to study biology/botanical ecology at the University of Salzburg. That way I can best combine competitive sports with my studies. I train around my schedule of classes. During the first year at the university, my parents rent a little house south of the city for us three kids: Gerhild is studying at the Pädak (University of Education) to become a teacher and Volli is training with the SSM Salzburg/Rif, a school for dedicated young athletes that combines academics and training, in track and field.

In the first semester, I hardly miss a student event. Life as a student is just too new, too interesting and too compelling. I don't want to miss a thing. During the first winter in Niederalm, I make lots of flat little loops in Hellbrunn Park just outside Salzburg with my cross-country skis; that's all there is room for. On the public bus from Niederalm to Hellbrunn, people stare at me as if I were an alien, with my skis in hand. But I want to be the best, and it doesn't matter at all how people look at me. I dream about belonging to a team, people who think like I do and understand me, about a coach who guides me, and about sharing my goals. I feel like I'm in a no man's land, not really at home anywhere.

Often I run to lectures and home again. The route always leads me over the Hellbrunner Berg, one of the Salzburg hills, at the foot of which lies Salzburg's Hellbrunn Zoo. I always look forward to this stretch. I run between the old lions and the Przewalski's horses, and usually at a time when I'm the only one there. Especially in the fall, when the leaves of the trees glow in lots of colours and I hear the fallen leaves rustling under my feet, I enjoy the running very much. I always try out new little side paths, and soon I discover a trail that leads me directly to a dead end above the wolves' pen. More and more frequently I'm drawn to this path – barely visible for others walking through the forest – and observe the wolves from above. I often slip into dreaming and philosophizing. How much sense does it make to keep this pack in the zoo? Such a small enclosure for eight wolves. Yes, they can hide themselves and withdraw from the curious gaze of visitors, but they can't retreat from the other members of the pack or just wander around. I don't know very much about wolves yet, but I do know that to tolerate their conditions in captivity, their will must be numbed. Like most of the other animals, too.

And yet I like going to zoos, wherever I am. One time, I was in the zoo in Seoul, South Korea. I was there as part of the Austrian women's marathon team, which had been invited to a big relay marathon along the 1988 Olympic route. A major international cosmetics company (!) took on enormous costs to invite the many athletes from countries all over the world – I will never forget the tiny women from Malaysia, who all ran barefoot and consumed mountains of little sausages, even at breakfast – or the roadblocks during our competition in the middle of the metropolis of 8 million people (at that time). And at the end of each leg, each runner was handed a towel with the logo of the cosmetics company to wipe away her sweat. It stank so strongly of chemicals that I threw it away immediately.

Seoul is so loud. Day and night, thick smog hangs over the witch's cauldron where civilization seethes uncontrolled. In all of the nine days we are there, I don't see the sun a single time, not even the sky. During the race we have one lane of the road for ourselves; alongside it are millions of cars, bumper to bumper.

After a few days, I have to get out of there. And having become curious about what life is like for the South Koreans, who seem so disciplined, I want to have a look at their zoo. Over the years I've developed the theory that you can say a lot about a society's values based on their zoo, their relationship to nature and what understanding they have of the various animals. I often think of a statement attributed to Arthur Schopenhauer: the way a society as a whole treats other species is an important indicator of its degree of civilization. Yes, I have to see the zoo. I go to the next subway station. The trains are endlessly long and come every 30 seconds. I squeeze into a compartment. Stoic faces surround me, and finally I've found a place where I'm the tallest person! I'm also the only blonde non-Korean. The zoo is far outside the city, generously designed, and you can glide horizontally over the entire compound in a long gondola. The enclosures themselves are small, simple, and more showcases than species-appropriate. Only the aviary for the beautiful native birds is enormous. Right next to it live two polar bears. Concrete below them, concrete behind them, concrete all around them. They just stand there and shake their heads from side to side, completely withdrawn into their living nightmare. The bears are there and yet not there. No one takes an interest in them, no one understands them, no one seems to recognize their needs. Their spirit is in a no man's land.

It's appalling. When I get back to the hotel, I'm immediately called to see the event organizers. It is not desired that I simply set out on my own to do something. Forgive me, but the trip to the zoo told me more about this society than a bus tour organized down to the last-minute detail, for which we have to be standing at the bus stop a full half hour before we get on the bus.

No, that is not my world. Nonetheless, or maybe precisely because of it, this trip is extremely eye-opening. Because I have experienced that free thinking and free will have no part in some cultures – even economically advanced ones – and aren't even desirable. Even the big bears suffer from it.

The Salzburg Zoo is almost idyllic by comparison. In fact, the quality of habitat there per square metre of enclosure is surely one of the highest in Europe, if not worldwide. But the available area is much too small in every zoo. Wide-ranging animals, which the large predators are, suffer the most.

I can never stay at the wolf enclosure for very long, because my time is strictly limited by my training. I am usually five minutes late for class, and then leave five minutes early again. Later, when my siblings have finished their schooling in Salzburg, we give up the little house in Niederalm and I live with my parents in Radstadt again. In the winter I have practise in the mornings, and then I have to hurry to catch the train to Salzburg – not infrequently Mutti hands me a lunch through the window of the train already in motion. In Salzburg I hop on the two-gear bicycle that's waiting for me at the Salzburg train station and rush to class. Afterward I do the whole procedure in reverse so I can fit in another round of training in the snow in the late afternoon at home.

Gerhild is also a good cross-country skier. She joins the Austrian student squad and immediately loves its atmosphere and semi-professionalism. Through her contacts I am also asked if I'd like to join. Yes, absolutely! The members share both of my passions: cross-country skiing and being a student. Wonderful. I participate in the first round of training. Finally I have like-minded people around me. In February the Austrian Academic Championships take place in Hall, near Admont. I'm allowed to go. It will be my first race in four years, since I became the Austrian champion in my age class the year I was at Stams. Four years without any ranking, without any indicators. I'm extremely tense. Will I come in last? Will all my dreams fall apart today?

Even before the race begins, it's clear that – thanks to our coaches Peter and Luggi – the team from Salzburg will win the prize for having the most fun. I have never laughed so much in my life as in those three days. And I relax a little. The morning of my race, however, there are so many thoughts racing through my head: How many hours have I motivated and tortured myself? How many tears have I shed from sheer exhaustion and desperation? How many social opportunities have I denied myself to preserve the chance that I might some day get where I want to be? How realistic is this whole thing anyway? Where do I stand? At the time, I define myself almost exclusively through my athletic performance, something that hasn't been put to the test a single time in four years.

Three, two, one – go! I start. And ski with everything I've got in me, all that I've built up through the years of painstaking work and under difficult circumstances. At some point I overtake the first skier; the climbs are easy and I even have enough reserves left to make a few powerful strokes over the crest and into the descent. I win the race and only then realize just how much this victory means to me. I am completely astonished and even more relieved. From that point on, everything happens very quickly. After a few summer training camps with the university's national team, the following winter I start for the first time at the Austrian Ski Federation's Austrian Championships. As a skier in the junior class, I stand on the podium every time in the senior category with older, more experienced skiers. The juniors' coach, Hermann Wachter, calls me over after the championships and says, "Gudrun, the World Junior Championships in Finland start in a month. I'd like to take you along. I think you have good chances of being in the front of the pack in the 15-kilometre race." At that time in Austria, that means placing in the top ten or 15. Through my lonely training I improved my endurance above all by going long distances; in combination with my still low weight, I'm not as well suited for the short, explosive sprint races. Fifteen kilometres is the longest distance for the juniors. I'm eagerly looking forward to this. The Austrian women's cross-country team consists of exactly two participants. In addition to the Czech-born Lucie Ptacek, I am the other 50 per cent of the team. To participate in the world championships in a country where Nordic sports are practically a religion is a dream come true.

In the athletic village I sit at the same table as Katerina Neumannová, who will later dominate women's cross-country for many years, winning several world championships and Olympic medals, and follow the first international successes of "Goldi," Andreas Goldberger, who is later an Austrian ski-jumping hero. My 5-kilometre race is terrible, as expected. I concentrate on my favourite distance, the 15-kilometre free-style (skating) race. I start the race as number two. Ahead of me is a German woman, Anke Schulze; no one knows yet that she has a huge career ahead of her. I'm a little frustrated that I never see her face during the race – she started half a minute before me. Nonetheless, I hear Hermann at the edge of the course shouting excitedly, "Gudrun, you're having a super race, you can be in the top ten! Give it everything you've got!" Which I do. And I cross the finish line with the second-best time of the first two competitors. But as more and more skiers finish, the significance of my achievement becomes clearer. Later Olympic winners in this race, including Canadian Beckie Scott, line up behind me. At the end of the race, Katerina Neumannová beats Anke Schulze. I come in 12th and feel like a champion. As I travel back to Austria, my suitcase nearly bursts, it's so full of newfound motivation. That was my first whiff of the rarefied air of international elite athletics. And it smelled mighty fine. I've hardly unpacked my suitcase and I'm already a member of the Austrian team. I find myself training alongside people I idolize, all with several years more experience than me: Maria Theurl, called Mary; Cornelia Sulzer, called Conny; and Jutta Mainhart.

In Austria, cross-country skiing is a humble sport, overshadowed by the great Alpine ski disciplines in terms of recognition and support. Sponsors and good coaching are in short supply. Achievements in the international scene are in the bottom half of the field. This is a Catch-22 cycle that is only broken when Walter "Woidl" Mayer becomes the head coach. A former winner of the famous Vasaloppet in Sweden, the Wimbledon of cross-country skiing, he brings a breath of fresh air to the national squad with his unconventional training methods and his sarcastic humour. Under his leadership the men become world class, with the historic high point being the world championship title in the men's relay in their own country, at the Nordic World Ski Championships in Ramsau, Austria, in 1999, and the Olympic medals earned by Christian Hoffmann, Alois Stadlober, Markus Gandler and Mikhail Botvinov. At the same time, the women's team is only half-heartedly supported by the ösv (Austrian Skiing Federation). Mary is the first to face the consequences and leaves the ösv. She focuses her attention on the Worldloppet, the world cup of ski marathons, and soon wins the overall world title. Cornelia seeks and finds her success in mountain biking and mountain running. She leaves behind a vacuum, in which Wolfgang "Pisti" Pistotnik builds up a young women's team. After a few years, two cross-country skiers emerge as the frontrunners: Renate Roider and me.

We qualify for the world championships in Thunder Bay, Canada. I am 23 years old and this is already my second world champs competition in the seniors category. The world championships take place every other year. My first was in Falun, Sweden, in 1993. As one of the youngest participants there and the fledgling member of the Austrians, I debuted in the mecca of cross-country in the 30-kilometre distance with a 24th-place finish. Jutta and Mary, who flew in later, were either not in top form or sick, like half of the Austrian men's team. As a result, my 24th place was the best result for the Austrian cross-country ski team at that world championships. Considering my tender age and inexperience, I'm completely satisfied. I can build on this. As a whole, however, the world championships in Falun are the nadir of Austrian cross-country skiing. Coaches are fired. And the ÖSV, spoiled by success in the alpine disciplines but also in jumping and more recently even the combined events, recognizes that it has to make changes. That's when they hire Walter Mayer – a good decision, because from that point forward, nothing is left to chance anymore. A house in Ramsau, the fulcrum of cross-country skiing in Austria, is rented year-round, and Walter's wife Gerlinde is appointed the legendary team chef. The medical care is optimized and the media professionally included. With his smooth comments, Walter becomes a favourite with the press and brings a new kind of ease to the team, which he uses as a front to implement aggressive training, cleverly hidden. All of this is for the men's team. We few obstinate women are an afterthought.

At the FIS Nordic World Ski Championships in Thunder Bay in 1995, the men's team experiences their first successes. Renate and I, on the other hand, have no dedicated trainers. The Austrian cross-country team rents its own house for the duration of the races. I miss the international flair of the athletic village that I found so exciting and motivating the last time. I feel neglected and uncomfortable when I observe the intensive efforts of the cadre of people dedicated to the men. I feel like I'm in a no man's land.

My boyfriend of many years, Michael "Michi" Grossegger, himself a trainer, follows us to Canada and brings my wonderful dog Sorro; only then do I feel a little more comfortable. But even the two of them can't make up for what I experience as the official ski team's indifference toward us women. To make matters worse, after we used the wrong wax in the first races, the two of us are portrayed by the media back home as tourists at the world championships. I'm glad I only find out about this after I return to Austria; this snub would have frustrated me too much.

In response to the trainers' indifference, I place 21st in the showcase race and miss the top 20 by 1.4 seconds. At this time, the Russians, Italians and Norwegians are in a class by themselves. However, the entire world championships will go down in history as the "diesel championships." We are in Canada, which for me has always been the country of pristine nature. The moment we arrive, all the athletes are given coupons to get drinking water from any store in town, for free. You can't drink the tap water, it's too contaminated. Everyone drives a car here – everywhere, even to the grocery store just around the corner. And most disgusting of all, the snow is brownish yellow. Greetings from the big paper factory. We feel the intensive industrial pollution under our feet with every step. The contaminated snow makes our skis very slow. This is my first impression of Canada.

Woidl, however, the consummate tinkerer, finds a solution for us: diesel. Before the next men's race, the Austrian trainers throw rags soaked in diesel fuel in front of their athletes' skis. It turns out to be the best combined results for the men's team. This world championships ends with mixed feelings.

For me, I know just one thing: I want out of the ösv. These days in an airless space have completely drained me mentally. If not even the ösv takes the slightest interest in our accomplishments, who could possibly care about what I do?

My world falls apart. Why am I following my heart, anyway? Can I afford that luxury in today's world? And especially when my heart doesn't give a fig about my status in society? Who cares about my athletic passions – what good is my training in biology and my passion for nature conservation to anyone? How insignificant am I?

There I stand in the country of my dreams, drinking water out of canisters, cleaning the polluted snow from my skis, and have to acknowledge that my many, many hours of training and deprivation hardly find any recognition at all.

Then Michi takes me in his arms. "Hey, you, don't be discouraged. You have to believe in yourself and invest in yourself. I'm counting on you. Come, train with me and my juniors group. My guys are at just the right level of performance for you." No sooner said than done. From now on I train with the Austrian juniors. Finally I have an enjoyable and motivating setup. Among the people I train with are Christian Hoffmann, Christoph "Sumi" Sumann and Daniel "Meso" Mesotitsch, all of whom will become world-class contenders. And I'm the inverse of the rooster in the henhouse. Michi believes in the same kind of innovative approach to training as Walter. In addition to rigorous training, activities like tightrope walking, canoe rides, chopping wood and even horseback riding are part of the program. Nothing like this has existed until now. Creative highlights are surely the slide boards, which are officially invented two years later and introduced to the aerobic studios of the world as a new fitness hit. By that time we have already slid holes through countless old socks and tested the entire contents of the cleaning supply cabinet of a cleanliness-obsessed housewife: what is the best lubricant for the plastic mats on which we glide from side to side for hours? For some inexplicable reason, our version of this exercise never becomes a big trend.

Something else that unfortunately doesn't become a big trend in Austria is providing some measure of security for elite female athletes in marginalized sports, in which you earn too much to die but too little to live. While the men are employed in organizations such as the Austrian armed forces, the police or customs, more or less "for the training," such options don't exist for women. (The Austrian armed forces were only opened to women for the first time toward the end of my athletic career.) My sponsors for many years were my parents, and the strategy was "spend as little as possible." There I had a double dose of luck: Papa supported me by always encouraging me, sometimes driving me to training locations or picking me up, or waxing my skis at night. But I felt most supported by his calm pride in my achievements. He gives me the unique satisfaction of bringing great joy to someone I love so much.

And I live in a region that offers excellent training conditions all year round. I don't really have to travel to a training camp and live in hotels there. Fall is the time for training on the Dachstein

Glacier. Half the world comes here; I just have to drive half an hour. Alois Stadlober, who lives 300 metres away from me as the crow flies, often takes me along on the glacier; sometimes Walter Mayer. I don't officially belong anywhere but am allowed to participate unofficially everywhere. I occupy no man's land once again – but in its unconventional way, this is even advantageous. I have the freedom to take my required courses at the university in Salzburg and still train at a satisfactory level parallel to my studies. You have to take new paths to make progress, and in order to leave tracks behind you. Sometimes the paths lead through no man's land – and sometimes you might even find you belong there.

ON EQUAL FOOTING
WINTER 1997

I throw my arms up in the air. I've just crossed the finish line of the biggest cross-country event on the North American continent, in first place. I've won the American Birkebeiner for the second time now, following my victory last year. I love the hospitality of the people here; the rolling course through the dense Northwoods of Wisconsin, home to wolves, is also very appealing. Everything about this race is perfectly tailored to me. At the mass start, the elite women are grouped in our own wave; that means we are allowed to start two minutes after the elite men and two minutes before all the others leave the starting line, a big advantage. We don't get lost in the crowd of strong male skiers and thus can have our own women's race. It still happens that the best of us women catch up to some of the elite men ahead of us. This is a skate-style race and the groomed trails in the forest are quite narrow in places. Passing is very difficult. But every time, something happens that is incomprehensible for us European female skiers. As soon as the men hear us coming up behind them, they call to each other, "The ladies are coming, get off the trail!" And then they make room for us. I think about the hot-blooded jostling for position during European mass starts. Highlights are the Marcialonga in Italy and the Engadin Ski Marathon in Switzerland. Both are extremely fast skate-ski races with a lot of prize money. At those starts, the elbows fly and you hear the cracking of fragile poles breaking all around you. But even at the mass starts of mountain running races I always notice that quite a few men don't appreciate being overtaken by a "weaker" woman. Many of the ambitious weekend runners have a personal goal: be faster than the fastest woman. In a mass start, a few minutes after the starting gun goes off, the men are typically ahead, but the longer the race lasts, the more of my male colleagues I pass. Is it because men simply have more power and thus get away from the starting line more explosively than women? Or is it because they overestimate themselves and then have to ease off?

The fact is that more than in any other type of sports, women come closest to the performance level of men in endurance disciplines. We are born endurance athletes. Pregnancy and birth require a lot of stamina and patience, as do years of childrearing or the millennia of being responsible for gathering berries and other food. We have great strength in us. The she-wolf reminds us of this.

This year there is a world premiere at the American Birkebeiner. For the first time in the history of the Worldloppet, the prize money for the women is just as much as it is for the men. I receive a cheque for US$7,500. It's a huge amount of money for me, even if I have to send half my winnings to the IRS. What I am most excited about is the organizers' recognition of our achievement. But this milestone doesn't last long. Lots of men complain to the organizers about this – in their opinion – unjust equal treatment. In the following year the fastest women once again have to forgo prize money.

Tartu Marathon, Estonia. The Worldloppet circuit has only included a stop in the former Eastern Bloc for a few years now, since 1994. Tartu is an emerging sports centre a few hours south of the capital city of Talinn. I have been invited there, along with Mikhail Botvinov, a former Russian who is now an Austrian citizen, and our trainer, Michi. We reside in a brand-new, super-modern hotel, so new that it isn't even finished yet. Just before its completion, the owners had a run-in with the Russian mafia, who supposedly burned down the entire building, and so it had to be built a second time. Welcome to the East.

This race has its own flair. The international elite athletes mingle with the many locals, who conquer the 63-kilometre stretch on wide, heavy wooden skis. Mikhail, who is dominating the Worldloppet, wins again.

And I am able to take first place for the women. At the awards ceremony, a big electric company appears as the main sponsor. Mikhail stands before a mountain of expensive entertainment devices including a giant television, a video camera and top of the line speakers. I stand before a heap of household appliances such as an egg cooker, a hand mixer, an iron and a vacuum cleaner. The last one I give to an Estonian woman right away. Taking it home on a plane would have cost me more than it's worth. I understand the message to be: "We want to lighten the burden of your work, woman, at home where you belong."

Near the end of every Worldloppet season is the highlight: the Swedish Vasaloppet, the longest of all the races, 90 kilometres from Sälen to Mora. It is the greatest cross-country competition of them all. Just like every Indian aspires to bathe in the Ganges River sometime or every Muslim hopes to make a pilgrimage to Mecca, anyone who wants to be a real cross-country skier wants to race the Vasaloppet at least once. The whole country is caught up in the excitement. The festival lasts an entire week with several different races, including the Tjejvasan, a race just for women, in the middle of the week, and a short 30 kilometres.

But it is the featured race on Sunday that hundreds of thousands of people follow live on radio and television, and at which the Swedish king has his own box near the finish line. Ten thousand people stand along the course. The race is limited to 15,000 participants, and every year it sells out immediately. Fifteen thousand skiers means 30,000 skis and 30,000 poles that all move out of the enormous starting area within the same instant in the early morning grey. Most of the skiers have already been standing at their starting spot for two hours by then, trying to start as far toward the front of the pack as possible.

It's cold and dark. To make the waiting more bearable, colourfully dressed aerobic ladies hop and jump on three high, wooden platforms alongside the several hundred–metre long starting area to loud, pulsing music and animate the freezing athletes to stay in continuous motion. We have the privilege of a starting wave reserved just for the elite skiers, so we can take our places in the last minutes before the start. Once Michi has the fabulous idea to rent a mobile home, in which we spent the night in the big parking lot right in front of the starting area. I am enjoying my breakfast in the warmth while more than ten thousand skiers have to do aerobics right outside the door. But a half hour before the race, I have to go get into starting position too.

The starting gun echoes above the enormous mass of people. Everyone immediately tries to move out as quickly as possible. It will be half an hour before the main pack has gotten under way. The race is in the classic style, so everyone propels themselves out of the starting area using the double-pole technique, a stretch with a slight incline. This gives men with strong upper arms an advantage. After about 3 kilometres, however, the tracks come together and at the same time the first hill begins. Suddenly the field is established. There is jostling for every position, even if it's nothing significant for the men near me. The leaders are already long gone. But I'm stuck in the field – like all the women. Whatever. I take part in the Vasaloppet three times, and all three times I miss the podium by one place, or a few hundred metres. Still, I'm very satisfied. While the women who win always train specifically for this race, I've already put my legs through hundreds of kilometres of racing, almost every weekend a long-distance race in a different place, each between 50 and 78 kilometres long. Not to mention the flying and time differences. Only once does it get under my skin. That time, if I hadn't urgently needed to make a brief pit stop behind a bush shortly before the finish line, I would have stood on the winners' podium. But instead I watch the award ceremony for the first three finishers from the spectators' perspective again, and again I cannot believe my eyes. At the biggest and most hallowed cross-country race in the world, the male winner receives not only hefty prize money but also a new car or snowmobile, and is showered with lots of other things to boot. The champion can practically take home one of the pretty young women in traditional Swedish costume handing over the prizes, while he's at it. Fair enough, it's an enormous accomplishment. Then the female winner is recognized. She too is the best of her gender, and she also had to ski the 90-kilometre course. She also trained hard for years to reach this point. She gets a sewing machine. As the woman in fourth place, I get a set of kitchen knives and a picture book. It fits well with my collection of Estonian kitchen appliances. But not with the valuation of elite sports in the 20th century.

My successes in mountain running and my distinctive path in the sport of cross-country skiing make me a good fit with the athletic profile of a start-up energy-drink manufacturer. Although I'm a relatively small fish, thanks to their support I am able to afford to continue my path and successes. The atmosphere is always personal, and when I visit the company the second question is always, "How did you do in the races?" But the first question is always, "How are you doing?"

The Österreichische Sporthilfe, an organization that supports Austrian athletes, creates a special fund for sports not represented in the Olympics, which reimburses me for training camps and certain other expenses. At this time there is no social safety net or insurance for athletes like me. This is my own pursuit; it is my own decision to do these things. And thus the consequences are my own responsibility. But at times I am very frustrated, so much so that I sometimes think I should enter the Tartu Ski Marathon again so I'll have a completely equipped kitchen for my career as a housewife. It would be the more acceptable lifestyle.

That it doesn't come to that, at least for now, is due to a happy coincidence. This is my third World Mountain Running Championship, taking place this time in Edinburgh. Yes, you can really run mountains in Edinburgh! The course takes us over King Arthur's Seat, an extinct volcano right in the city. Our Austrian team is well positioned again. After the superb successes of the previous year, mountain running is finally getting a little more press coverage. Among others, the head sports editor of the most widely read tabloid in Austria is there. My meeting with him ends with me switching to the running club LCC Vienna. Their president, Dr. Peter Pfannl, believes in me and becomes my supporter for many years. The Radstadt Ski Club and Salzburg Regional Ski Association take over some financial expenses. And the company whose skis I use pays premiums for wins that vary according to the size of the race. All of this brings in a little money, and so I eke out a living.

NEW TERRITORY
SUMMER 1992

The Japanese guest is delighted with the breakfast omelette. I'm relieved. I have only been working in the small, elegant garden hotel in Salzburg for a week. But it is understood that a guest's wish should never be denied, and anyway, challenges are opportunities for growth. It is August and the Salzburg Festival is under way; the city is filled to bursting with tourists. Gerhild has been helping out here for a while. We clean the rooms and place a chocolate Mozartkugel on the guests' pillows. One time, we both run on the Untersberg in the evening after work and sit together on the peak as the sun sets, with the hectic city far below us.

The next day I'm called to the phone at the hotel. "Hey there, Gudrun, it's me, Franz Puckl, from the Kitzbühler Horn race! Was an amazing record you set there last week." I grin. *Yeah*, I think to myself, *it is pretty amazing how well it went for me*. My appearance at the most widely recognized international mountain run had some similarities with the making of the omelette: no experience, but rising to the challenge! And most important, it ended well, in every possible way. I made it to the peak in good form not in spite of but because of the extremely inhospitable conditions on the upper stretch, with sleet and cold wind. When I feel the elements on my face, it mobilizes extra reserves of energy within me. I love storms and rain, while other runners freeze in that weather. Capricious weather is my ally. It contains so much energy, and I'm always able to draw a little of it for myself.

Recently I've started mountain running in the summer, in addition to cross-country skiing in winter. In the summer of 1992 I win my first real race at Kitzbühler Horn. All at once I'm known in the mountain running scene. "Gudrun, do you have time next weekend? 'Cause the world mountain running championships are going on in Susa, in Italy. We've got a good women's team, but Isabelle just got sick on us. We need one more for the team competition. And you ran so well." And so on and so forth. Franz likes to talk and has a typical "crackling" Tyrolean accent. But to summarize the phone call: I'm supposed to start at the world mountain run championships next weekend. And the result: I immediately quit my summer job, and four days later I am sitting in the team's van on my way to the Susa Valley. During the drive I ask my experienced colleagues what's important to know about the world championships, in a nutshell. In a kind of spoken rap, the essential information about the event is shared with me: women's 7.5-kilometre loop course, about 30 countries at the starting line. The Italian women's team is the favourite, the French are not bad and the British are represented by several teams. The sport is so big in the UK that each region sends its own team. We arrive in Susa late in the evening. The next morning it's pouring rain. Then a thunderstorm rolls in. The miserable weather continues overnight, and on the day of the competition the start is delayed by several hours due to another thunderstorm. After noon the rain finally stops. The entire racecourse is thoroughly soaked; the narrow paths have been turned into rivulets. We start anyway. I know nothing about the course, about my competitors, about any kind of strategy. The only thing I know is that every step counts.

Every time I run past coaches and spectators standing along the course, they scream, "*Ale*, *ale*, Isabelle!" Soon I notice that I'm in the lead, but this Isabelle must be right on my heels. It makes me crazy not to be able to see her. I feel like I'm being hunted by some ghostly phantom that I can't shake but can only feel on the back of my neck. At the peak the racecourse turns downward along the fall line toward the finish. On a slippery, wet, grassy ski slope, the course is staked out like a kamikaze mission. Now I'm really glad I'm so naive. I'm wearing my cross-country shoes; I didn't own anything else at the time anyway. But they have long spikes on the soles, which isn't typical for mountain running. Now I'm going to show this Isabelle how you run down a mountain – ideally without thinking about it too much. I have to concentrate completely; on terrain like this, every step can be your last. And so I never turn around to look behind me. The finish line comes into view. At the same time, the screaming for Isabelle is getting louder and louder and more fanatical. I stride across the finish line, and the loudspeakers announce: "World champion, winner of the World Mountain Running Trophy: Isabelle Pichler." And then it occurs to me. I was substituted for Isabelle Pichler on such short notice that they couldn't change the list of participants. I am Isabelle! But more than that, I'm the world champion!

Twenty years old and world champion in an endurance discipline that demands more experience and tenacity than almost any other sport. As icing on the sweet cake, our women's team also takes home gold, thanks to the excellent performances of Anni, Sabine and the young Cornelia. The men, including Peter Schatz, Helmut Schmuck, Florian Stern and Markus Kröll, also have an excellent race. These are the golden days of Austrian mountain running.

But Michi reminds me that mountain running exacts its pound of flesh, and I still want to achieve my goals in cross-country skiing. So in the next five years I compete only in certain carefully selected mountain runs. Without my being aware of it, my years of training have been the perfect preparation for a different sport as well. In the next five seasons the many hours I've logged in powerful ski strides translate into a total of four World Trophy triumphs – the official name of the world mountain running championships at the time – and additional wins in the biggest mountain races in Europe.

Because I'm not training specifically for mountain running, and have little invested in it, I really have nothing to lose in these races. I develop a laid-back attitude that has extremely positive results. Indeed, in addition to my all around intensive training, it becomes the most important factor in my success. Through this distinctly carefree approach, I even begin to find the joy in athletics that hasn't been very accessible to me before. The big distinction between the running and the cross-country skiing is simple: I've invested in one sport, and in the other I'm reaping the rewards for it. Later I observe this productive equanimity in the best cross-country skiers in the word. And I am convinced that it's one of the most important elements of success in any endeavour.

Cross-training, in other words training in multiple sports, lateral thinking, and determining my own path all belong together.

These accomplishments in mountain running are not my first experiences with track and field, though they are certainly my most successful. Thanks to my brother Volli's connections to the Salzburg/Rif Sports Centre (a top-notch facility associated with the university but also available to the public), soon after I become a student I join the Salzburg Union and train under Hannes Langer for the 3000-metre race, cross-country, and later half-marathons too. He doesn't have it easy trying to make my automated long strides and arm motions a little more suitable for track. Taking part in a "running school" at the age of 20 leaves me wondering how I managed to ambulate at all in my first two decades of life. But the training has phenomenal results, not to mention the atmosphere at the sports centre, where there is a steady stream of weekend athletes and elite athletes, soccer players, swimmers, rowers, runners, ski jumpers – the list of disciplines is long. In addition to me, Hannes also works with truly great talents like Laurin Madl and Tanja Burits. Laurin is powerful and always in a good mood. Tanja is young, pretty and a 3000-metre specialist. Together we travel to the high-altitude training centre at St. Moritz in Switzerland. The purpose of a change in location is not only that the change of scenery does the soul good but in this case to practise in the more difficult conditions at higher altitudes. The body responds to this stimulation by generating more red blood cells, which transport oxygen molecules from the lungs to the rest of the body. It's a classic trick of all endurance athletes. I share a room with Tanja. She tells me about her big dreams and athletic goals; they are lofty, but she can achieve them. The next summer, Chinese female athletes shatter the world records in the 3000- and 5000-metre races in their home country. Tanja's world implodes. She never recovers; struggles with bulimia, then drugs. One morning she is found lifeless. Cause of death: overdose.

For a long time Tanja accompanied me when I raced. Every step counts. Also for you, dear Tanja.

Laurin suddenly has to fight a tumour in his brain. And loses the fight. Every step counts. Also for you, dear Laurin.

Just before the new millennium Papa dies. He too isn't able to beat his cancer. Every step counts. Especially for you, dear Papa.

I can't understand why some people apparently aren't rewarded for their wonderful, marvellous being.

My steps grow slower. Their meaning has become more questionable to me over the years. In 1998 I officially end my active career as an athlete with four World Trophy victories in mountain running, the Worldloppet cross-country ski championship, many individual wins in international races, and more than 25 Austrian championship titles in cross-country skiing, mountain running, half-marathons and cross-country running.

WOLF SPIRIT 7
OCTOBER 2005

A few days after the operation, Phil and I pick up Mutti from the airport in Calgary. They've removed my tumour. Cut open my skull in the shape of a horseshoe, then separated and removed the growth in the left temporal lobe. Put my skull back together and attached it with staples. I didn't even lose a hair. The next day, I lay in bed attached to a morphine infusion at Foothills Hospital, Phil at my side. Apparently friends even came to visit, but I don't remember. What I remember very clearly, though, is the night before the operation. First the surgeon, Dr. Ian Parney, with the informed consent forms, from which he read aloud all the dangers of the upcoming procedure. I had to swallow hard. And I had to sign. In the evening my friends Mike and Shelley came to visit and brought me a soft blanket to cuddle. I didn't want to let them leave; I was afraid of being alone with my agonizing thoughts. It was late when they finally went home. Everything was dark and quiet. Now I was alone. The place where I spent my last night before this decisive operation wasn't even a real room, just a compartment. Gloomy. I saw tubes, nothing human, except my security blanket. I stared into the dark – and then a warm feeling of comfort and confidence came over me. A powerful peace overtook me and let me sleep deeply.

First thing in the morning, I was wheeled to the operating room. The surgical nurses took off my jewellery, the wolf amulet from my neck and my rainforest ring from my finger. It was difficult to part with these two things. The nurses asked me about my work with the wolves and as I answered I fell fast asleep.

It was a successful operation. Dr. Parney could remove all the visible tumour tissue. But it is my brain, and in the brain you can't operate *in sano*, in other words cutting away a generous margin in the surrounding healthy tissue. And it is an aggressive kind of tumour. All of this requires further therapies and months, maybe even years, in which I will live between uncertainty and fear, but also with constant hope.

Two days after my operation, I am back in Canmore, get out of bed and have a burning desire to go to the river. The Bow River is the lifeline of the valley and runs for the most part freely, even through Canmore. It divides itself into tributaries and forms islands and other structures. The wildlife, including grizzly bears, as well as the human population, love the trails alongside its meandering course. It's very early and no one is out and about yet. At a bluff a short path leads upward. I want to go up there. To prove to myself that it's not so bad. I can still do this. On hands and knees I slowly crawl upward; speed has no meaning anymore, only the goal of reaching the top. I make it, and during the moment in which I look down at the river, a herd of elk cross it. I will never forget that sight. It motivates me to make my rounds along the river every day from then on, through brush and over beaver dams, stepping over wolf scat and observing coyotes, elk and bald eagles.

Nahanni is always with me. My gait is very slow, and I grow weaker and weaker the longer the chemo and radiation treatments last. But the joy I derive from this walk becomes greater and greater. At some point I have to work my way up even the smallest incline with all my energy and with the help of my arms. Nahanni stays by my side, going at my pace, standing, waiting. Without a leash and with no impatience. She adopts my rhythm as hers. She reminds me that time is just something added on, nothing essential. And that nothing matters but the next step.

When I am able to move into the apartment in Calgary organized by Mike, I just relocate my daily walks a hundred kilometres downriver. Here too the Bow River flows freely, through the big city. My apartment is only two minutes from its banks and a ten-minute walk from the cancer clinic at the hospital. Everything is perfect.

It is December. The days are short and it's already very cold. The plentiful Christmas lights I would usually find terribly kitschy are truly illuminating for me, in the literal sense of the word. A neighbour, Yolanda, introduces herself, and she starts to bring me super-healthful food once in a while. She's also a physiotherapist and comes a few times to give me a massage. I can count the days on which I'm alone on one hand. My friends from Canmore and Calgary have an actual schedule to keep track of who is with me when. It's wonderful. The constant distraction works wonders.

By myself I can't read a book; even watching television is too taxing for my eyes, which the radiation has made incredibly tired.

I spend hours listening to the radio, healing music, and audio books that my friends bring me. Sometimes we play simple games. Vanessa always has some kind of entertainment along, whether it's nail polish or beads that we put together. But most of the time, I just let them tell me what's going on at home, or sleep.

One night, when I happen to be alone, a powerful storm kicks up outside. It's the chinook, the warm wind that blows down over the Rockies. Like a greeting from the mountains it descends, shaking and rattling my window. Finally, it pushes the window open. The refreshing wind rushes through the room and fills it with energy, a contagious vitality. I jump out of bed, intending to close the window but instead end up standing in front of the open window for a long time, breathing in the night air. It's as if it wants to call to me, "Come along! You belong outside in nature, in life!"

"Chinook, can I give you something to take with you? All the bad stuff in my body that doesn't belong there? There, you have it. Please take it away."

It seems like the wind is racing through me, through my head. Cleaning it. And dissolving everything that's unnecessary into thin air. Then it becomes calm and I close the window. And fall asleep again feeling lighter.

The Wisdom of Grey Owl

PRAIRIE LIFE

PRAIRIE WINTER
WINTER 2003-2004

Riding Mountain National Park lies like a wild island in the middle of an ocean of grain fields and meadows and grassy plains on the prairies of Manitoba. Ironically, it has the shape of a giant pistol pointed westward. On 3000 square kilometres of gently rolling hills, dense boreal conifer forest alternates with lighter poplar woods and extensive grasslands. Between them, lakes, grasslands and deep ravines round out the landscape. In addition to hundreds of species of birds, large herds of elk and moose, as well as bears and wolves, roam the protected area.

When I arrive at the Moon Lake warden station, it's bitterly cold. Typical prairie winter. Park Warden Glenn and his wife Lorraine greet me warmly and show me my lodgings for the next several months. The little park hut is right next to their house and Glenn's office. There's a horse barn behind it, and that's the extent of the buildings at the Moon Lake station. It's at the north entrance of the national park on a – relatively – big road that connects the town of Dauphin, about 20 kilometres north of the park, with Wasagaming, the main settlement in the park, which lies to the southeast. Dauphin will be our main source for shopping and borrowing books, and the starting point for our observation flights. Astrid, a doctoral candidate from Norway, is heading the research project on wolves in Riding Mountain National Park.

Eight wolves have been outfitted with radio collars. Patty helps us find the wolves in this vast landscape. She is the owner of the mini air carrier at the Dauphin airport. Astrid and I take turns flying with Patty in order to locate the collars' signals from the air and thus find the animals. I usually love to fly; it reveals so many hidden treasures of nature, and only from above do you get a true overview of the landscape. Connections you hadn't realized before are revealed. It's often important to see things from a certain distance and from a new perspective. So I generally like to fly. And I also usually enjoy the sight of wolves. Nonetheless, I am usually pale as a ghost when I get out of the little Cessna propeller machine, and I forgo a big breakfast when I know I'll be flying that morning. Flying at low altitudes and the tight circling in on the signals is nothing for a weak stomach, no matter how skilfully Patty flies. But it is a new and thrilling method of tracking wolves. The main line of questioning in our project is: to what extent do the wolves, in spite of the isolation of the park in surroundings drastically changed by humans, still have the opportunity to interact with other wolf populations? In order to find that out, I often drive to the nearest woodlands, Duck Mountain Provincial Park, to the north of Riding Mountain.

Duck Mountain Park is 70 kilometres away as the crow flies. Seventy dangerous kilometres for the wolves through open farmland inhabited by people. Can the wolves from Riding Mountain, members of one of the most mobile and adaptable wild species in existence, still navigate this distance through territory hostile to them in order to draw fresh genes from the wolf population in the provincial park? Astrid needs genetic material to find out, as much as possible. And once again I'm promoted to chief poop collector. I drive thousands of kilometres back and forth in search of the mounds and cover hundreds of kilometres on skis – as a Norwegian, this is of course no problem for Astrid, either. More of a problem is that Dauphin is such a small town that there isn't a single café that's open during the winter. I compensate for this lack of cultural offerings by taking guitar lessons. Unfortunately, the teacher would rather hear himself play than his student. And so my skills as a guitarist remain deeply buried under the thick snow of the prairie.

Astrid is highly intelligent, a genius with languages, and has a good sense of humour. In the Norwegian tradition, she sets candles all around, and we are never without a pot of hot coffee. Even today she is one of my most reliable friends. At the end of the winter, we have spent many cold days skiing, but more important, lots of lovely hours together as friends. We survive winter camping at −30°c or create the "Riding Mounting Witch Project" together – these are bonding experiences. The latter took place at the end of a canyon. We happened to find an antler from what was once a stunning stag captured in the frozen ice of a stream. A little later another one, then ribs and more elk remains. All told there are remains of 12 animals, and it's clear: this here is a cool wildlife criminal case. When we climb up the steep slope, we recognize the strategy behind it. The ravine takes a sharp turn at this point, which results in a narrow patch of forest that comes to a point. The individual trees here have taken a beating; they all bear clear traces of repeated life-and-death battles. I can only shake my head, once again impressed by what the wolf packs have come up with. They have quickly learned to take full advantage of their surroundings, and as a perfectly coordinated team they have driven the elk toward the slope; the ravine took care of the rest. Fascinated, I stare down into the depths at the work of highly developed social intelligence, the work of the wolves.

Unfortunately, however, they can't always escape from the so-called intelligence of humans. I follow the signal of a female wolf with my antenna; it's very close by. I cautiously continue walking. Maybe I'll find her with a new pack, because she was actually captured and collared in a different area and has left her home turf for the time being. All of a sudden, the signal is gone. I think I'm dreaming. This can't be. I continue in the direction in which I last heard the "peep peep" and reach the boundary of the national park. Along it runs a gravel road. I stand there facing the suddenly wide-open landscape with lots of raised hunting blinds lined up along the border, hesitating. A rickety blue pickup truck approaches; the driver pulls up next to me and opens his window. He points to the antenna in my hand.

"I just drove her to my place. Was in my snare trap." I sigh deeply. "Hop in, you can take her with you. Saw her collar, of course. Part of a national park project?"

"Yes, she was."

He lives right nearby. His little wooden house is full of mounted animals. Proudly he shows me a lynx with her three kittens. All on a shelf on the wall. His wife makes coffee. I ask if I can make a phone call; I want to let the park ranger know they should come get me, Nahanni and the wolf here. My car is parked heaven knows where.

"Where is she?"

"Behind the house, on the pile where I keep all the coyotes over the winter. Most of them are frozen solid when I find them. Just need to wait for spring when they thaw and I can skin them. There, there she is."

Her face is frozen in a grimace of pain; there's a broken piece of branch in her blood-smeared muzzle. Her hind legs are deeply bent, and her outstretched front legs indicate that she tried in vain to defend herself from the slow, stealthy approach of death due to the wire noose around her neck. No, it's not a pretty sight, and one of the low points in my work studying wolves. A very realistic scenario that we have to face if we want to learn and understand. Someday I would like to understand how people can sleep well after doing something like that. What goes on inside the heads of people when they lay the snares, what they feel when they skin the animals and let the bodies rot in piles. Someday.

The elderly couple are very nice; they tell stories and share many of their treasured trophies on the wall and important experiences with me. But understanding? I cannot understand them. Even though trapper Franz emigrated from Austria a long time ago, and we share the same mother tongue.

The prairie surrounding the park is crowned by a seemingly endless sky, a broad horizon that promises openness, foresight and a genuine generosity. And that's how the real residents of the prairie are. The space that surrounds us also shapes us and our character. Even if many farmers aren't thrilled by wolves, they accept them, in part because the wolves' selective hunting helps reduce the transmission of tuberculosis from infected herds of wild elk to their cattle. The wolf serves as a kind of health police. Some cattle ranchers here even view the wolf as their partner, because they have too many beavers on their land that flood large sections of pasture. Others are proud to have active wolf dens on their property. And then there are those who don't care one way or the other. And some just hate wolves.

Astrid creates a tolerance map that indicates the attitude of the landholder toward wolves. At the end of the study we can see that this tolerance has more influence on the distribution of wolves than any other factors or criteria in the landscape. Where there are people willing to live with wolves, one finds wolves. In places where people have decided wolves are not desirable, they stand very little chance of survival. At least not in a landscape that is as easily accessible as the prairies. This realization makes me stop and think. It's further proof of the extent to which we influence, shape and rule our environment, and how dependent our environment is on our capriciousness. How helplessly it is subjected to our will. Because in spite of our power to change things, far too often we humans don't perceive the responsibility that is so closely connected with that power.

The Jeep makes its way through the snowstorm, but the snow-covered road hasn't been distinguishable from its white surroundings for quite a while. Thank heavens the roads are 99 per cent straight here. On the radio I hear a program about the spring Flower Count taking place today in Victoria, the capital of British Columbia. Famous for its favourable climate, each spring the city takes the opportunity to flaunt its warm weather while much of the rest of Canada is still buried deep in snow. A great example of Canadian humour and how diverse the country is.

Just yesterday, thickly bundled up, Astrid and I took an extensive snowmobile tour with an old ranger in the Duck Mountains. I was so cold I almost fell off.

The locals are an interesting mixture of European immigrants whose ancestors were granted a section of prairie to cultivate at a giveaway price, and new arrivals who come to the area looking for peace and quiet and a place to unfurl their creativity. Thanks to Paul, who has lived here for years and wrote his dissertation here, I meet many wonderful people. An internationally successful journalist/photographer couple that turned an old school into their home, for example; or the owner of the little 60s-style roadside restaurant that serves the best burgers in the region; environmentalists who are full of life; intellectuals who find enough space for their ideas here. The prairies are big enough for everyone.

And there is space for valuable friendships. Astrid occasionally has to spend some time at the university, and then I work alone. One day I drive to the warden station at Baldy Lake, at the opposite end of the park. Blair, the park warden stationed there, comes toward me from a long way away to greet me. He and his wife Deb don't often get visitors here at the end of a long, lonely road. They live with their cat and their horses in a small clearing on a rise with a wonderful view of the park's hills. When I see the two of them, something like "love at first sight" happens. Blair impresses me with his calm, content demeanour and his mischievous humour. His ways remind me a lot of Charles, someone I worked with in southwest Alberta. Later I find out that the two of them are good friends. A few weeks later Blair shows me in the lab how to dissect white-tailed deer and examine them for a type of BSE, or mad cow disease. Deb immediately displays her warm, welcoming nature. After my exploratory tour, they both invite me in for coffee. Deb pulls my favourite coffee from the shelf. It's only roasted and sold in the Rockies. "Where did you get that?" I ask Deb, astonished. The coffee is just the first of many things we have in common. Deb is still my best friend today.

Both of them originally come from the foothills of the Rockies, and they have a house in Canmore. They want to be in the mountains again, and in fact, a year after we first meet, Blair takes a job in Banff National Park and Deb works for the big heli-skiing company Canadian Mountain Holidays (CMH), which was founded by an Austrian. That allows our friendship to continue to deepen, because after this winter season in the foothills and again the following winter, I go straight back to Canmore.

At the end of February, Astrid needs to return to the university for good. In the thawing landscape I take several long tours, first on skis, then on snowshoes and finally in rubber boots. While I am camping one night, my tent is surrounded by the pack in that territory. I hear their steps all around me, then a howling from atop a hill. I step outside the tent, but I don't see anything. Nahanni stays right by my side. She can probably sense the size of the pack. The next day, I find fresh tracks everywhere and spend the day searching for the den that I think must be nearby. Thick brush in nearly impassable terrain makes the search fruitless. And on top of that, I have a toothache.

When the toothache rapidly gets worse, I have to evacuate myself as quickly as possible the next morning, because there is already too little snow for a helpful warden with a snowmobile but too much snow for a horse.

After a long march I arrive at the next warden station, exhausted, and drive immediately to the dentist the warden recommends. He has to pull my badly infected tooth, and I'll have to deal with complications that result from it for years to come.

When the national park is engulfed by masses of thawing snow at the end of March, I spend a few days at Brandon University to learn first-hand the process of extracting genes from wolf scat and analyzing them. I'm able to stay with the geneticist. During the day we work under artificial light, surrounded by machines and tubes, on the analysis of samples that have been collected over the past months. In the last step of the process, you shake the glass test tubes and suddenly fine little threads form in the cloudy liquid. With my own eyes I can see the book of life: the DNA strands found inside the nucleus of every living cell that regulate all life on Earth. It's an unbelievably fascinating sight!

With this fantastic image in my mind, I pack up my things and again drive westward, toward the mountains. The vast fields are underwater and dotted with millions of migratory birds. They are taking a rest along their long spring journey northward. Their presence transforms the flat prairie into a three-dimensional land-scape full of life.

NEIL YOUNG
WINTER 2003

"And take the warmest clothes you have. It's 30 below out there and incredibly windy," Erin advises me at the end of our phone conversation. That's not a lot, I think, and pack my anorak on top, easily accessible. Then Nahanni jumps in the truck. We're on our way to Saskatoon, Saskatchewan, the "Paris of the Prairies," 700 kilometres east of our starting point in Canmore. Even before the Rocky Mountains completely disappear from the western horizon, I have to pour an entire bottle of motor oil into the engine. But I've stocked up and forgive the Toyota. It has a good excuse: it's old.

In spite of everything, I'm still proud of my first Canadian vehi-cle and enjoy the feeling of freedom it affords. Without your own car, it's difficult to impossible to get around in Canada. The infra-structure is designed around cars, and everything is far apart, even within a town. There are few sidewalks and bike paths compared to Austria. And the Canadian Pacific Railway, the CPR, transports almost nothing but freight from one end of the country to the other to the big international harbours in Vancouver or Thunder Bay. If you're in pretty good shape, you can hitch a ride with your bike on a laden freight train. And, in the West, if you have lots and lots of money, you can book the luxury route, the all-inclusive train trip from Banff to Vancouver. That costs more than my truck. But it is less nerve-wracking. Again I pour in a whole container of oil. "Come on, girl, we only have to make it as far as Saskatoon." In Saskatoon the car belonging to the research project awaits me.

Now I'm driving with Nahanni through the prairies, the icy cold wind whistling through the gaps in the windows, my com-fort be damned. Nahanni lies tightly curled up on the passenger seat. Snowdrifts make the border between the road and fields invisible. On the radio, they correct the current temperature downward. Infinitely long and straight, the road heads east. If my steering wheel were to freeze in this position, I think, it wouldn't even be a problem. Or the turn signal. You don't need either one of them here. Lyle, my good friend with at least 20 lives, comes from Winnipeg. He knows each of the three trees on the thousand-kilometre-long stretch between the mountains and his home in Winnipeg, the capital of Manitoba.

He used one of his lives somewhere out there in a cornfield. Whenever he's driving through the prairie, he mounts a kind of provisional music stand on the steering wheel and reads entire books. But one time, he fell asleep while reading and woke up in the middle of a field. He didn't know where the road was and had to wait a long time before a car drove by so he could figure out which direction the road ran. I, on the other hand, play Neil Young the whole time. He's from Winnipeg too. Like Lyle and an ex-roommate of Phil's and mine, Jason, the best mountain runner in Canada. Nothing is flatter than Winnipeg, and the highest point there is a restored landfill. For years, that was his training ground.

When you drive through the prairie, you just have to listen to Neil. I begin to comprehend how deeply this expansiveness can mark people. Anita, Paul Paquet's wonderful wife, comes from the Provence region of France and now lives with Paul in the prairie village of Meacham (population less than one hundred). A few houses, two churches and an old wooden grain silo, that's Meacham. For a long time the two of them had a house in Canmore as well. Anita is fun loving, intelligent and ready for any adventure. She is a gifted artist. And precisely because of that, because she has an eye for little things, a knack for the details, she has always been an extremely successful wolf-scat locator.

She always felt crowded or pressured by the mountains. "You know, Gudrun, I just need the space and the huge sky. They inspire me. This is the only place I can really be creative." With every kilometre I drive, I can relate to her statement more and more. I've never seen so much sky. Out here it's not only above me, like in the mountains, it's also in front of me, next to me, behind me; it's all around me. I could actually say it the other way around: I'm in the sky. And instead of angels serenading me, Neil is singing. I like it.

The province of Manitoba neighbours Saskatchewan to the east. Along with Alberta, these are the provinces with the greatest areas of prairie, those seemingly endless tracts of grasses in the heart of North America, with rich soil that made the first settlers dream of prosperity. The settlers established one farm after the other. They came from all over the world, and especially from countries that were plagued by famines in the second half of the 19th century, like Ireland or the Ukraine. Today's prairie farmers claim they are a tough folk. And everyone would have to agree. When the first farmers settled here, they benefited from a few decades with exceptional rainfall. The new arrivals understood this to be the normal climate. But the conditions that are actually typical of the region soon returned. That means dry, hot summers and frigid, polar cold in winter. Winnipeg is often the coldest city in Canada, sometimes rivalling places farther north. When the weather changed back to normal, the new farmers struggled with crop failures – as much as 100 per cent. Many of them stayed in spite of this, but others gave up. The government looked for successors to work the wheat and canola fields.

Every time I look out an airplane window as I fly from Europe to Canada, I recognize the prairie immediately. Today it looks like a gigantic checkerboard divided into thousands and thousands of square of greens and browns of all shades. The original grasslands that so impressed the first settlers have all but disappeared. Its cultivation was too easy. But the eager farmers didn't reckon with one important factor: the hefty prairie winds. Hot and merciless, they dry out the cultivated land and year after year blow away the valuable humus soil. The prairie turf that once protected the land has long since been plowed, loosened and eroded. There are no more great herds of bison, which provided natural fertilizer. Today, endless monoculture farms ingest huge quantities of artificial fertilizers and pesticides provided by the global corporation Monsanto: leaders in a modern version of playing with fire; experts in genetic manipulation. Grain is their guinea pig, the prairie their experimental laboratory. For one, Monsanto changes the genetic material of the grain so that plants are now hybrids. That means new seeds are not capable of germination and can't be propagated by farmers. Now farmers have to buy new seeds from Monsanto every year. But this is only one aspect of the company's coup. Grains, especially canola, are manipulated to such an extent that they tolerate high concentrations of the all-around pesticide Roundup – also manufactured by Monsanto – quite well. So farmers make another purchase from Monsanto, this time a higher potency of Roundup – and in generous quantities. Farmer rebellions are not tolerated. And where the bison herds once grazed, the agri-mafia are now raking it in.

But now everything lies under a snow-white covering. Even at these temperatures and with car troubles, for someone like me from the Alps it's incredibly beautiful to travel through these wide-open spaces. The infinite sky melds with the earth somewhere out there. The longer I drive, the more I find myself in a Zen-like state of mind. I've never been so pleasantly relaxed behind the wheel. Beautiful, these silvery-blue colours everywhere.

After more than 600 kilometres and eight hours, I reach Saskatoon. Erin is waiting for me in her little rental apartment. Together we drive to the university where Erin is a student. She wants to write her master's thesis about the wolves in Prince Albert National Park (PANP). And of course, Paul Paquet is her supervisor as well. The national park is 200 kilometres north of Saskatoon. Its nearly 4000 square kilometres are covered with boreal forest in the north, aspen parkland in the south and the transition zone between them in the middle. Twenty per cent of the park is water. The large lakes are already frozen solid when I arrive. The land rolls gently, the maximum altitude difference not even 250 metres. On the way to my new home for the next five months, we stop in Price Albert for a big shopping trip. I will be staying in lodgings in Waskesiu, the only town in the national park. It lies on vast Waskesiu Lake, and I'm told it's overflowing with vacationers in the summer months. I see nothing, absolutely nothing, that would suggest this: the businesses are locked up, the gas station abandoned, all the hotels shuttered. Only the Haywood Hotel is still open, and the little post office next door. In the winter the vacation resort belongs to the employees of the national parks, the elk herds and the wolves. And starting today, a little bit to me, too. There are places you arrive at for the first time and feel immediately at home. Prince Albert National Park and Waskesiu are among those places for me.

I love the stillness and the feeling of family there. The park employees get together in their time off to play ice hockey or darts. They exchange news, of which there isn't much. The elk stand by the tennis courts and especially like to bed down on the golf course. Then we finally see some action. The park custodians equip themselves with hockey sticks and chase the elk off the precious lawn because the animals come in droves and paw through the snow until they reach the juicy green grass. Besides, the cows have their calves with them, and they would quickly get used to the golf greens, which would be a big problem in the summer months. Hoofed animals can attack people. They are often underestimated, or people get too close. At least the employees have something to do. It doesn't get any more Canadian than this.

THE ASPEN PARKLAND WOLVES
WINTER 2003

My task is simple: gather as much wolf scat as possible from as many different areas in the park as possible. Paul Paquet has lent me his wolf research car to help me get around. My dilapidated truck can have a long winter's rest parked outside my apartment. The red wolf Toyota with manual 4-wheel transmission is perfect – so perfect that I buy it from Paul at the end of the season. Between now and then lie countless kilometres on the snow- and ice-covered roads of PANP. Pretty soon I can identify the tracks of wild animals, and even recognize their hair, while doing 50 kilometres per hour. I prefer to gather hair instead of scat, because the latter tends to be a stinky pancake stuck firmly to the road. Pretty soon I borrow the appropriate gathering tools from the park's road maintenance crew: a pickaxe and a spade. I use these implements to scratch many hundreds of these pancakes from the asphalt.

Wolves love to wander along roads, often for many kilometres. And when they come fresh from a kill, their scat is usually very dark, extremely pungent and quite thin. Through Erin's study, Parks Canada wants to find out how many wolf packs or how many individual wolves there are in the park. To do that, you analyze their DNA. My GPS, in which I save the location of each sample I collect, tells us exactly where the individual wolves we've identified are spending time. Even more important, genetics helps us understand the extent to which the protected area is able to fulfill its mission of maintaining healthy genetic diversity in the population. Around the park in every direction the wolves continue to be ardently pursued by hunters, trappers and cattle ranchers. Can the wolves still exchange genes with the animals in the less impacted North? This is an important line of questioning for those hoping to encourage long-term preservation of diversity in the species. What would our planet be without the many and diverse manifestations of nature, after all? Impoverished, terribly impoverished. And poorly equipped for changes of all kinds.

There are two methods you can use to find out what the local wolves eat. You can sterilize their scat and wash it, because after all, what goes in must come out again. Then you can take your time examining and sorting all the undigested parts of the prey. The task of scat washing is beyond the pale, but the remains are like the contents of a treasure chest. Astonishing stuff comes to light, from intact jaws or hooves of deer to bear claws, and of course lots of bones, teeth and hair. We used this technique, especially with the coastal wolves. The second method isn't as precise as the first but more elegant: you compare the proportion of stable isotopes – especially nitrogen and carbon – in the hairs or other parts of all the possible prey animals that are available with that of the wolves. Through model calculations, you can figure out the proportions of each nutrient in the prey. Both techniques start with the same material: scat, or poop, as they say in Canada.

Each morning I use a map to plan a new tour to search different areas for scat. Then I make a quick stop at the park office, which is always filled with the scent of freshly brewed coffee. Staff let me know if there are any new wolf reports, and I inform them about my approximate route for the day. I always carry a mobile radio with me, too, but in this cold and with all the dead zones in this region, you can't always count on it to work. Then I'm on my way, most often on cross-country skis; this sport just won't let me go. Erin's Uncle Herb owns a big hotel in Waskesiu. It's closed in the winter, but Herb is also the head of the Malamute Nordic Racing Club in Prince Albert. It isn't long before he's standing at my door, as excited as a kid that I've landed here, and he can lend me ski equipment to use while tracking. The landscape and especially the enormous frozen lakes are really ideal for it; the equipment less so. At the end of the season, it's ready for the trash bin. It was embarrassing for me, but in the very first week, the cold was so intense that the boots became so brittle that they fell apart. But Canada is prepared for such emergencies and millions of other hardships: there is always duct tape. The answer to every catastrophe, it is a wide, silver tape that sticks to everything, is extremely tough, easy to tear off, and the number one article for all outdoor activities. To transport it, I just tear off a few metres from a new roll and wrap it around my hard-plastic water bottle, the second essential item for the outdoors.

For the rest of the winter, I follow the tracks of the wolves for many kilometres in my duct-taped cross-country ski boots. On wide, slow, heavy skis and with two heavy poles. When I stay out overnight, I'm also pulling a repurposed child's sled, heavily laden and prone to tipping, behind me. But I've never enjoyed cross-country skiing so much in my life. This kind of movement is perfectly suited to this terrain, to me and to the wolves. The long stretches bring me into the deliberate rhythm of the frozen landscape. Even the sounds are frozen, and often the only thing I hear for hours at a time is the swishing of my skis on the raw, cold surface of the snow. It's as if all of nature lies in a blissful, deep slumber under the thick blanket of white.

Today there's not a breath of wind, and I'm standing with Nahanni at the edge of a lake in the backcountry. Nothing. I hear absolutely nothing. Does such a state still exist on our planet today? I close my eyes and strain to hear something, anything. In vain. There just isn't anything. The land around me is filled to capacity, every centimetre of it, with silence. I just stand there and take in the complete absence of sounds. Unfortunately, this doesn't last very long. I can hear a humming in my own ears. They aren't used to having nothing to process.

Nahanni runs alongside me, stopping now and again to test the wind, roll in the snow with abandon and then sprint toward me again. When I gather wolf scat, she curls up in the way huskies and wolves do and watches attentively with one eye until I complete my work. She leaves me to do the dirty work from a safe distance. But soon I decide I don't like this. "Nahanni, you should do a little something to earn your keep." I've decided to train her to be my wolf scat detecting assistant. It's quite simple: I take a filled sack from the field house with me and deposit it – well-wrapped and marked – in the freezer. Every evening the sack serves an important purpose: I put Nahanni in the bathroom for a few minutes and hide it somewhere in my apartment. Then I let her out and she has to find the wolf scat, which she always does quickly. Such are the games wildlife biologists play on long, lonely winter nights.

The days are very short in winter, and so it's not unusual for me to forget to turn around when I should. When that happens, Nahanni leads the way home with the white underside of her upright tail. During the daytime, dogs and wolves see about as well as we do. But in twilight they outperform us. The reason is the tapetum lucidum, a mirror-like surface behind the retina of many animals that reflects available light, providing the light-sensitive retinal cells with a second chance at photon–photoreceptor stimulation. This enhances the animal's ability to see in low light. All species of wolves are also much more sensitive to movement than humans, especially at a distance. I don't need to say much about their hearing and their excellent sense of smell. Both are legendary. Wolves can perceive the howling of their own kind from 8 kilometres away and smell prey up to 2 kilometres away. Especially in the dark, I'm always aware of how poorly equipped humans are for sensory perception in comparison to other predators; in a biological sense, that's what we are. When the light falls, I place my full trust in Nahanni and her senses, and she always brings me reliably back to the car. Just like we do, dogs – and as I have personally experienced, wolves – and most other highly developed animals sense when you trust them. I have no idea what exactly they perceive; maybe we are simply more relaxed and make broader movements, or maybe they know it through their noses, which gather different scents from us than when we approach them with mistrust. Or is it the mirror neurons I've already mentioned (see page 86), which I find so fascinating? Or a little of everything? I find that the most plausible explanation.

We humans have a tendency to think in discrete categories. This was criticized by the Swiss pedagogue Johann Heinrich Pestalozzi at the end of the 18th century, when he applied the term "fragmented knowledge" to the school system, which conveys information without context and thus completely neglects interconnected, contextual thinking. Particularly when it comes to wolves, we all have to admit that we only know fragments of the truth. But the information we have should at least be comprehensible, verifiable, and based on evidence. Here in Prince Albert National Park, I again have the opportunity to add a few more pieces to our body of knowledge about wolves: multiple times I find kills near the shore on the ice of the lakes. The hunting sequence seems to be routine. The pack approaches the lake together, fans out to encircle a section of forest, and forces an animal that happens to be in the woods toward the ice. As soon as the prey steps onto the slippery surface, the wolves with their rough pads have it easy; the hoofed animal slips up for the last time. (Only once do I find the actual site of a kill to be more than a kilometre from the shore.) After the deed is done, the wolves hang out for hours on the open ice, feeding, sleeping, playing and being mobbed by cheeky ravens. Sometimes so long that it actually gets boring to watch them. What a luxurious feeling that is.

The killing sequence itself can be read quite well in the snow. Where do the wolves turn toward the lake? Where do they encounter their prey for the first time? How far from there until the first drops of blood colour the snow red? How many wolves are directly involved in the hunt? Where do the others join them? Is the prey already weakened by then; can it still jump or does it just wander aimlessly through the brush? Even if the wolves are already lying around the kill site with full bellies or most of them have already taken off, until the next snowfall the tracks in the snow tell the precise story – to anyone who is prepared to look for them, see them and try to understand them.

The main prey of the PANP wolves is white-tailed deer. On the last day of work before Christmas, the park staff invite me to their communal Christmas celebration. Since it doesn't begin until 11:00 am, I go check the southeast shore of Waskesiu Lake in the morning. Soon I discover the fresh tracks of the entire local pack. Eight wolves have recently patrolled the access road parallel to the shore, then turned abruptly toward the lake. After crossing a patch of woods, their tracks lead onto the ice. I don't even have to look at the tracks in the snow; the cawing of the ravens is already calling it out to me: "Here is a kill! Here is a kill!" And when I step out of the forest at the shoreline, I see a dead deer lying on the ice less than 100 metres from the shore. Nahanni is already standing next to it, wagging her tail. Wow, thanks for the fabulous Christmas present, she's probably thinking. Not a chance; it belongs to the wolves. I look over my shoulders to both sides. The wolves can't be far away; the liver and all the inner organs are still intact. That's what they always eat first. I'm sure I didn't disturb them and chase them away; Nahanni would have let me know that. I look at my watch. The Christmas party is about to start. Reluctantly, Nahanni and I move away from the kill, but she's quickly helped herself and torn off a foreleg. Her expression leaves no doubt: this has to come with us in the car. Well, all right. It's almost Christmas.

The party is very casual and warm, and for the first time this year, it gives me the feeling that it's Christmas; it also gives me a touch of homesickness for Austria. At home in the Alps, the weeks leading up to the holidays are bound up with more cozy, charming traditions than probably almost anywhere else in the world. Even if those weeks are usually anything but calm, they still make me feel a sense of belonging and appreciation. In Canada I haven't heard a single church bell ring in eight months. Everything blinks, and an entire holiday-decoration industry makes a killing by selling Christmas kitsch every year. The quantity of holiday decorations set up on lawns and houses is hard for a European with a modicum of taste to swallow. But this little celebration with the people who are interested in and working for the same things I am helps a little.

When the party slowly comes to an end, I'm right back at the southern shore. I cannot believe my eyes: the deer that was still intact less than three hours ago is gone. There's nothing left but a few bone fragments and traces of blood. Shortly after I found the kill, two park wardens saw the wolves 15 kilometres farther to the east. They must have come back those 15 kilometres, eaten the entire deer and moved away out of sight in the same time it took me to drive a little way, eat turkey and Christmas cookies and sympathize with the young daughter of two wardens – a bad case of stage fright led to her piano performance being cancelled. The kill site fits perfectly, for me, with the meaning of Christmas: what a gift! And that's exactly what I'm thinking to myself now. I stand at the site of the kill, and all I see before me is the still frozen outline of the deer's body that was lying there, still intact, not long ago. No signs of the deer at all. A bizarre sight. Spooky, unreal. Wolfish. The efficiency of wolves is often astonishing.

THE LAST BREATH
WINTER 2003

"But then I shot her anyway." I heave a deep sigh. I had just felt that little spark of hope flare up in me, the slight smile on my lips, the nodding of my upper body in agreement. The rancher's living room is very cozy. A classic Canadian log house just outside the western border of Prince Albert National Park. Through the big windows I see his cattle grazing in the pastures. There's lots of brush between them and the mixed forest of aspen and conifers farther out. I received this rancher's address from Erin. She had learned he might have wolf DNA samples at home. One could say this guy shoots wolves. Lots of dead things hang on the lovely log walls, from moose and caribou and elk to black bear and wolf. He talks freely about his profession as a rancher and the challenges of his work. The land is hardly suitable for it. The climate is extreme, the earth acidic and wet, and there are enough wolves that they are a problem for his herds. Like many of his ilk, he earns a little extra in the winter by setting traps. The fur industry isn't what it used to be, but he still makes a small profit. I ask him about the wolves.

"Yeah, I get them pretty often. But the beasts are clever, very clever. You have to do everything just right. Pay damned close attention when you're setting up the trap. Can't leave any scent at all behind, and I have to simmer the traps in my special brew for days so they lose the smell of iron."

"Have you ever observed any of them?" I ask.

"Nah, you don't see them, only when they're dead, in the trap. That's enough for me. All I see of them are my dead calves." I listen to him calmly, let him take a thoughtful pause. Then he starts talking again. "Well, I once had a wolf in my trap, she was still alive. Her right front paw was caught. I can remember it well. It was a winter evening, really cold. When I got close to her, she wanted to hide from me. I loaded my gun. Then she sat up straight and howled. It was a really beautiful wolf, the snow made everything bright, I could see her clearly. I can still see the warm breath that came out of her mouth. You could see it in the cold air. Was an impressive moment. Really gorgeous animal. I hesitated before I fired ... but then I shot her anyway."

He couldn't jump over his own shadow.

ROYALTY
WINTER 2003

Prince Albert National Park is named for Albert of Saxe-Coburg and Gotha, the beloved husband – and cousin – of Queen Victoria, who ruled the British Empire at the time the nearby city of Prince Albert came into existence.

The food supply for wolves is also fit for royalty. In addition to many types of deer, they also eat beaver. The only source of food they haven't really tapped into yet are the bison, which have only been grazing freely in the southern part of the park for about ten years. I have found signs that suggest the wolves are starting to take an interest in the newcomers, but they probably haven't developed the right hunting technique for them yet. When you are suddenly confronted with a giant like that, you think very carefully about how hungry you really are. Bison are, after all, the largest land mammals in North America. I always keep a respectful distance from these creatures. I'm just not familiar enough with them to be able to interpret their body language. But at the same time, I've always enjoyed observing them – from a safe distance – roaming in nature. This species has been through just as much as the wolf and is recovering with great difficulty. A bison's size doesn't allow many of the things that help wolves hang on: their secretive lifestyle, for example, isn't something bison could imitate. And even more than the wolf, bison suffer from new competition: the domesticated cattle, which have claimed what were once their grazing lands. Today they can only live in the wild where people allow it, in national parks.

The only herd of plains bison that ranges freely in their original territory in Canada grazes in Prince Albert National Park. The twenty animals that were reintroduced here have increased to a healthy population of about four hundred. Because they roam freely, they often cross park boundaries, and as a result a regional management plan is required. They are the true royalty of the park. In addition to the plains bison, there are also wood bison. Both are subspecies of the North American bison, millions of which once lived on the prairies. The largest herd living in the wild is a mixture of wood bison and plains bison in Wood Buffalo National Park, over 44,000 square kilometres – more territory than Switzerland – on the border between Alberta and the Northwest Territories. It is a UNESCO World Heritage Site. All of these conservation efforts came too late for the mountain bison. It is already extinct.

The bison territory is in the southwest part of Prince Albert National Park. Tourists seldom venture there; the roads are terrible, making it difficult to reach. It's the realm of the heavyweights: the bison and Lloyd, "the King," as his warden colleagues call him. Lloyd almost lives the life of a recluse in his park guardhouse, except his neighbour, who lives a few kilometres outside the park, drops by for a round of cards every day. Otherwise the big old man takes care of his babies, the bison. He drives his snowmobile through the Sturgeon River Valley, where the bison like to hang out. When I meet him, he immediately pulls out a second snowmobile.

"Here. If you want to look for wolves around here, you'll need a snowmobile. Ever driven something like this?"

"Nnnnooooo, not for a long time." I've driven a snowmobile a few times in the Rockies, but I prefer to claim inexperience so I make a better impression, if it comes to that.

"Okay, it's easy. Here's the starter, here's the choke, you accelerate here and – oh, yeah – here's the brake. Come on, let's go for a ride." And he's off. It isn't long before we come to a little brook. Lloyd gives his machine some gas and simply jumps over it. So I also accelerate, and drive straight into a tree. Bang. Lloyd rushes over, has a look at the mess, and scratches his head thoughtfully. "Hmmm, well, that doesn't look good." The front of the snowmobile is woefully crumpled. I'm terribly embarrassed. But Lloyd stays cool. "Oh, well, I have to go to the office in the next few days anyway. I'll just take this with me. They haven't got anything to do in the garage in the winter anyway. We'll just tell them a story."

I'm glad it's taxpayers' money I've just plowed into a tree, I think to myself. From then on, I ride on the back of Lloyd's machine – until Nahanni, who runs along behind us, exhausts herself to the extent that she vomits. Then it's back to my roots. I return to what I learned: cross-country skiing. Now Nahanni and I can really enjoy the area for the first time. I breathe in the fresh, clear air, hear the ice murmuring, and once again see much more of my surroundings. We cross a large lake. Something black is moving in the distance. Nahanni has seen it too and immediately determines her mission. That thing has to be confronted. It's an otter, slip-sliding across the ice in its typical, entertaining way: hop, hop, slide along the belly; hop, hop, slide. Otters always live in or near water. In the winter, they need openings in the ice to have access to the water below it. This otter is a long way from such a hole out there in the middle of the lake. I yell after Nahanni that she should leave that poor animal alone. From a distance I see her nudging the otter, and I already see blood flowing. But then she jerks back and is in a big hurry to run back to me. I think the otter taught her a lesson about who's in charge around here.

AL DENTE
WINTER 2003

In Rome it's 21°C. Here in PANP it's –28°C. Elisabetta packs her suitcase, I my down jacket. She steps into the plane, I put on my skis. After about ten hours, she arrives in Calgary – at the same time, I fall into my bed in my little apartment in the national park, exhausted. Two days later, Erin turns into the driveway of the building where my apartment is, delivering Elisabetta. In the Italian way, Elisabetta immediately jumps out, waves to me and gives me a hug. As of that moment, I have an assistant. Elisabetta wrote her thesis about the feeding behaviour of the wolves living in the southern Apennine Mountains. Now she wants to gain some experience in a different country. Marco Musiani, a good friend and Italian professor at the University of Calgary, liked by everyone, connected us. I like Elisabetta immediately. She's the personification of Italian temperament. She brings some Latin warmth to the cold northern winter. Nonetheless, I put her on a pair of cross-country skis I quickly borrowed from Herb on day one. "Elisabetta, there's no way around it. If you're going to tag along with me, you'll have to learn how to ski." She's never had a pair of skis on her feet in her life. "It's just like walking with poles – then glide." As I look down at my boots held together with duct tape, I say, "...but with *this* equipment your technique won't matter, anyway."

Six hours later we return to the car. Elisabetta is grinning, although she's exhausted. I am delighted; she's been a tough cookie and was able to follow all my tips about her technique. Yes, Elisabetta will definitely be a tremendous helper. Very soon she's not only an assistant but also a friend who will go through thick and thin with me, and the best medicine to dispel loneliness. Finally I have someone to talk and laugh with, and to cook with in the evenings. There's pasta in every variation, but one thing they all have in common: they're cooked al dente. I don't like half-cooked noodles. Here we have a difference of opinion. But we quickly solve this fundamental issue: Elisabetta just takes her noodles out of the pot sooner. After a few months, we discover another point where our tastes diverge, which actually turns out to be an advantage. There are two interesting friends, male and near our age. I've been seeing Jeff for a while now, the older brother of a girlfriend from the Rockies, and we spend many hours together. Jeff has a friend, Greg. He works for the parks service. And how could it be otherwise: the Italian starts to see Greg regularly.

This makes the cold winter warmer and sweeter for us, and as spring approaches, Elisabetta and I start to change out of our old, torn anoraks from the second-hand store and our duct-taped ski boots (Elisabetta's didn't make it very long without duct tape either) after our work in the bush and trade them for light, flowery dresses. Jeff is head of the work crew at the Elkhorn Resort golf course, just outside the gates of the national park, and in winter he grooms cross-country tracks on a snowmobile for the guests there. He has more time now than in the busy summer. Life is good. The four of us take turns inviting each other over for dinner. Sometimes the European gals cook, sometimes the Saskatchewan guys. They tell us stories about their many joint canoe trips "up north on the Churchill River" and the "craziness" here in the park in summertime.

In the cold months before that, Elisabetta, Nahanni and I make several overnight trips into the backcountry. The wardens provide us with steaks and the keys to huts where we'll stay overnight. We both pull children's sleds behind us. The goal each time is to replace the weight of our very generously packed provisions – in addition to the enormous steaks, a big head of cabbage always travels with us, among other things – with wolf scat on our way back out. We recognize that there are more wolves and wolf packs in the park than previously thought. We celebrate that every night with a candlelit dinner of steak, pasta, coffee and cookies while a fire crackles in the little wood stove. Often we overdo it with the heating so that first the old iron stove starts to glow and then the entire hut heats up like a sauna. Then, late in the night and close to naked, we run out into the snow of the −30°c night. That cools us off fast.

In the beam of our flashlights, we read the wonderful "tall tales" recorded in the journals of the old wardens. We find them hilarious. Our laughter and the light from the hut penetrate the dark, cold night. The bags with the deep-frozen "wolf specialty" stay outside the door. They must not thaw; they need to stay "al dente," shall we say.

GREY OWL
WINTER 2003

Grey Owl was born in England in 1888 as Archibald Belaney. He died in Prince Albert National Park in 1938 as the "Indian" Grey

Owl – or Wa-sha-quon-asin, from the Ojibwa word *wenjiganooshi-inh*, which means something like "great grey owl." At the age of 17, he boarded the ss *Canada* in his home country and sailed to Halifax on the Atlantic coast of Canada. He soon forgot his original plan to study agriculture and instead worked as a trapper and wilderness guide in the northern reaches of the province of Ontario. There he met the Anishinaabe–Ojibwa First Nations, learned their language, married a young Ojibwa woman, and lived among them. Over time he claimed to be a Native American. After the First World War and additional marriages, he ended up at Ajawaan Lake in Prince Albert National Park with his 19-year-old wife Gertrude Bernard, a Mohawk–Iroquois woman who is also known as Anahareo, the name Grey Owl gave her. Anahareo convinced him to write about his wilderness experiences and his rich knowledge. He became so successful that he was even invited to give lectures in England and talk, above all, about his work with beavers, as a purported "real Indian." The noble Europeans stormed the lecture halls to see the "noble savage" and hear his beaver tales live and in person.

Elisabetta, Fiona and I load the snowmobile on the trailer of the Parks Canada truck. Fiona and her husband Adam are park wardens in Prince Albert National Park. Fiona is a wonderful soul, and all three of us are excited about this camping trip near Ajawaan Lake. The winter has already relinquished its harshness, and we're even setting out in T-shirts. The plan: while Elisabetta and Fiona drive ahead with the snowmobile to the little warden's cabin north of the lake, I'll ski to the cabin with Nahanni. First we have to get past the long, stretched-out Kingsmere Lake. The snowmobile ladies will travel along its eastern shore and I'll search for tracks on the western side.

I enjoy the first spring sunshine. The glistening crystals – billions of them – cheerfully reflect the sun's rays on the frozen lake. I breathe deeply and take the fresh air deep into my lungs. Gratefully, I feel the velvety warmth of the warm air. During the past months I've worn a cloth over my mouth most of the time to warm and moisten the air I inhaled with my exhaled breath. Otherwise the cold air felt like needlepoints in my bronchi, especially under exertion. I'm familiar with this from cross-country; if you have to breathe deeply at very low temperatures, it can burn like hell.

I continually have positive experiences with everything that I learned through high-performance sports. For a long time I thought I never wanted anything to do with that world again, wanted to get away from the image that kept me stuck in Austria. I wanted to devote my time and energy to something I find more meaningful, more important. Almost like Archibald Belaney gave himself a new identity as Grey Owl, I also wanted to leave a lot behind me and have nothing more to do with the often brutally egocentric approach to life in professional sports. I saw my last years in elite sports as more of a dead weight, as wasted time. Because my heart was already somewhere else and had been for a long time. Because in my early years as a wildlife biologist, athletics didn't mean anything to me anymore. I only thought about all the experiences in wolf research I would already have under my belt if I had chosen that path earlier.

I've never talked about my athletic career very much, but the consequences of it were clear even without a lot of discussion. It was always obvious that this new line of work is ideal for me, physically and mentally, precisely *because of* my past. Now my time as an athlete comes up again and again, but exclusively in a positive way. And I can only be grateful for those years of training.

I glide easily over the glistening lake, able to enjoy it thoroughly, and at the same time concentrate fully on the search for signs of wolves. Another benefit to my former life as an athlete is that I always have the full confidence of all my project leaders and directors. Elite athletes, after all, have a reputation for determination and a strong will.

Years later I hear a talk given by Steve Jobs, the founder of Apple and one of the greatest visionaries and most successful people ever, who died in 2011. He talked at Stanford University's convocation ceremony that year about "connecting the dots," about things and especially experiences that only gain their true meaning when you look back on them later. Their actual significance is only revealed in connection with other experiences. His talk resonated with me. I have experienced this myself.

Because it's such a joy to ski under the blue sky, I incorporate a few detours. Fiona and Elisabetta will make sure the cabin is cozy and make something delicious for dinner by the time Nahanni and I arrive in the evening, hungry and tired. My "catch bag" is getting quite full. For kilometres I follow the tracks of an entire pack across the broad expanse of ice. The tracks repeatedly show that the wolves take time to play during their travels; they also seem to have enjoyed the simple act of moving across the lake on the hard-packed snow. Slowly the sun sinks toward the horizon to the west; its rays are flatter and weaker now and take daylight with them. And quickly I am reminded that it's still only March in the North. I pick up the pace, although my legs are starting to feel all the kilometres I've covered on skis today. But the anticipation of the obligatory giant steak keeps me going. It's not far now to the northern shore. Now I see the opening in the forest that indicates the beginning of the trail to the cabin. Fiona and Elisabetta's snowmobile is parked right next to it. As soon as I step from the relatively bright surface of the ice into the forest, I can hardly see anything anymore. But I can feel how I sink into the soft snow, warmed by the sun, in spite of my skis. Oh no, I think to myself, it could still be a long way to the cabin tonight. In my imagination, that steak gets bigger and bigger. Slowly I fight my way through the mush and against the darkness. But I'm counting on my ally, the encroaching cold. It should hurry this time, please, and create a firmer ground for me. It's calm; only my steps and Nahanni's panting fill the forest. The steak continues to grow. The forest opens up to reveal a view of Ajawaan Lake. On the opposite shore, I can just make out the outline of a cabin. *That must be the cabin of Grey Owl, his wife and his beavers*, I think. What a peaceful setting. Out here you can still concentrate on what's important to you. No critical voices. The trees watch patiently, and the lake reflects and intensifies all dreams. The shore reminds you of the importance of continually starting anew. Yes, here you can follow your innermost purpose, or at least find it.

Suddenly I hear voices. They can't be coming from the cabin yet; according to the map it's still another 5 kilometres off. The fresh boot prints are not a good sign. Then a faint light shines through the trees, and soon I see the outlines of two bent figures. *No, please, dear universe, please – don't let it be what I fear. Don't let it be Fiona and Elisabetta!* Fiona and Elisabetta turn around. "Gosh, Gudrun, the snowmobile kept getting stuck in the melting snow. We're completely exhausted." The steak has now grown to the size of an entire cow. Together we tug and pull our gear through the deep snow in the dark forest. Eventually we reach the cabin, too tired for a steak even the size of a mouse. Nonetheless, Fiona immediately thinks to start the gas camping stove. At least a cup of tea. She fiddles with the starter and suddenly there's a "puff!" The old device explodes, and an enormous flame shoots toward the ceiling. Black smoke envelops the room, and we run to get wool blankets and snow. Hectically we throw both at the burning kitchen corner, with success. Other than large black spots on the wood walls and ceiling, no one will ever notice a thing. The cabin will be torn down in the coming months anyway.

The next morning the weather is once again ideal. While brushing her teeth outside the cabin, Elisabetta sees a wolf pass by. That determines our course for the day. I will follow the wolf while Elisabetta and Fiona survey a transect. We take our time with breakfast and packing up, giving the wolf a two-hour lead. Because I don't want to be chasing it away from me. It should do exactly what it would have done if we weren't here. When I set out, following its tracks, I already find lots of fresh deer tracks that cross the wolf's path. I even find the clear, heart-shaped hoofprint of a deer inside the paw print of the wolf; the deer is following the wolf. So much for the theory that prey animals always keep their distance from wolves and stay away from their territory.

I come over a crest and see a small lake at the foot of the slope. In the middle of the glistening ice, a black wolf lies rolled into a ball, sleeping in the morning sun. It's far enough away that Nahanni can't pick up its scent, nor the wolf ours. I have already neatly shovelled its fresh scat into a plastic bag. After this season of field-work is over, it will be brought to the lab and analyzed for remnants of DNA. The results will be a matter-of-fact combination of numbers and letters, destined for a chart. In the best-case scenario, it will give this wolf a unique identity and reveal who its relatives are. The decision makers and their advisers, the representatives of industry and the environmentalists will play with that information, interpret the numbers according to their own interests. For them it will always remain a number. For me it will always be this beautiful image of a wolf with all the additional information that can't be crammed into a table: its pristine natural surroundings, its trust in its environment, which it demonstrates when it curls up on this open expanse of ice, all alone, and sleeps tranquilly. This sleep might even be the difference between the success or failure of its next hunt. And above all, the non-verbal, emotional impressions of such moments. They always arouse something in me like a deep, dormant longing for paradise. The image before me is simply a black wolf sleeping on the open ice of a lake under a blue sky in the middle of a late-winter landscape. Just that, and yet so much more. For a few breaths it silences the longing in all of us to become one with everything that is. The lightness of the thought that all my duties and responsibilities are momentarily suspended, that is freedom in the moment. I am simply there. And part of it.

Moments such as these open the possibility to give up one's self in order to become open to our actual purpose. We have to preserve the potential for these moments for all of us. The wild places on our planet are the realm of the senses and emotions. The places that are healing, moving, and at the same time strengthen us. We have to preserve them. Before the last of them disappear.

In challenging situations I will often recall such moments as this perfect scene of the black wolf on the white lake, hold on to them like a life ring when I'm once again experiencing stormy seas in my own life. These memories fortify me for all future challenges. Little experiences with enormous impact.

In the evening I return to the cabin. Elisabetta and Fiona are already waiting in the inviting warmth. A fire crackles in the stove, and the steaks sizzle in the pan. Late into the night, the trees and creatures of the forest hear happy laughter from a little cabin – somewhere out there where life is still simple.

WOLF SPIRIT 8
OCTOBER 2005

The spirit of the wolf is with me and Dr. Parney. And the spirit of many, many friends and my family. During these six hours of operating they have all thought about me, prayed for me, sent me white light and positive energy. Whatever anyone wants to name it, it was with me and this concentrated positive energy contributed to the success of the operation. It was the first time that I could consciously feel thoughts as reality. It would happen many times again. Our thoughts are energy; they are real. And they are tied to time and place. Many people at home in Austria were with me just as much as all my Canadian friends.

It is the time of the secret, through which you can get everything you wish for. Again and again I watch the film titled *The Secret*, as a weapon against the doubts and the fear. The film is hope: I CAN get healthy again! And my Canadian friends are especially encouraging: "Yeah, Gundy, you're strong, you can do it!" It's like in a race. These cheers and encouragement and the vitality, my surroundings, it's all perfect. I live in Canmore, where there is an outdoor community second to none. It's a place for *lebenskünstler*, people who are masters at the art of living, people who are forging their own trails, believe in themselves. Those who think everything is possible and act accordingly. A healing place. Friends and people I've never seen in my entire life come and bring bright bouquets of flowers, tokens of good luck, audio books, or meals they've cooked. Winter is approaching and Phil travels for work quite often. Friends declare wellness days and paint my toenails;

we watch movies and they tell me what's going on outside my four walls.

I also receive lots of good wishes from Austria, most of them delivered through Mutti, but also letters and phone calls. All of them mean well. But something is different. The vibe of their words is more pitying and sorrowful. Succumbing to fate. Austrian. Slowly I understand why we call America "the land of unlimited opportunities." People believe in success and work toward success. Failure is not presumed; at most it's seen as a necessary stop along the way to success. Hope dies last.

And yet: why me, of all people? I ask this question exactly one time. Of Dr. Easaw, my oncologist. He answered with one word: "Destiny." Then I know there is no answer. And I never ask this mother of all questions out loud again. At the moment, everything seems pointless. Things couldn't be better in every aspect of my life than in the past weeks and months. So why now, of all times? When Gerhild and Phil and I visit a shaman, I don't ask the question, but I receive an explanation: "Gudrun, only people who can cope with it are singled out for this disease."

The disease is one huge question. Over time, though, the questioning is transformed into its own answer. And all the reasons why its appearance at this particular moment is illogical become the arguments for why it actually does fit particularly well in my life right now: in thousands of hours and situations, life has prepared me for this illness and given me all the reasons why I love my life so much as weapons for the fight against the cancer. Now I have to learn how to put them to use.

I don't like these aggressive expressions of war relative to my illness, and so I search for words that suit me. Soon I describe my irrepressible will to be healthy with the image of my inner wolf, my wolf spirit.

This life force possesses all the many positive characteristics of the wolves that make them, too, resistant to great challenges. In the stark world of the tundra I have experienced their irrepressible will to live; their kilometres of tracks in the deep snow of the

Rockies testified to their endurance and determination; the survival of a sick she-wolf in the coastal rainforest for years proved to me the presence of mutual support among wolves; the many choruses of howling animals sang of their powerful bond.

Yes, I have a serious illness, but I also have many highly powerful remedies:

- *my exceptional level of physical fitness and mental fortitude from my past in athletics;*

- *the many people who stand by me in thoughts or with actions;*

- *the successful operation and, later, special viral therapy; and*

- *my deep relationship with nature, in which everything seems possible – this was so distilled in my encounter with the coastal wolves that I know it is a gift, a tool and a mission.*

The Beauty Lies in the Barrenness

TUNDRA TIME

NEW TRACKS IN THE NORTH
SUMMER 2002

We call it "tundra time," the time in which we just sit around and watch. We're actually waiting, but in order to know when the waiting will have an end, we have to keep watching. Constantly and in every direction. It's incredibly hot. Hotter than I have ever experienced anywhere else on our planet, even though Paul and I are sitting somewhere in the Barren Grounds, not too far from the Arctic Circle. We are flown in by an Ekati Diamond Mine helicopter. It will pick us up again in a week and then take us to another wolf's lair. Hopefully the pilot won't forget us. When he has helped us unload, we stand next to our heap of camping gear and wave at the receding helicopter. *There goes our connection to the civilized world,* I think.

For five days our little camp with the two yellow dome tents has stood in exactly the spot where the pilot dropped us off – somewhere. As we flew in we scanned the nearby esker from the air for signs of wolves – and found some. That makes this area our home for a few days. Eskers are long, sandy end moraines, remnants of glaciers in subarctic regions that can extend over many kilometres. They are the preferred sites for the dens of tundra wolves, strategically located along the caribou migration routes. That's where the female wolves give birth to their young and the starting point for their hunts. As I sit there and scan the landscape with my binoculars at regular intervals, I can only wonder how the wolves here manage to stay alive. Rocks, stones and gravel, between them lakes, thousands and thousands of lakes big and small. In spots where a little humus has accumulated, low-growing plants add a little variety to the austere landscape. The precipitation rate here is that of a semi-desert, but what little rainwater falls gathers in the rock depressions and often leads to wet feet or long detours around the many swamps. The land is a part of what is called the Canadian Shield, an ancient bedrock formation that stretches out over 8 million square kilometres. In fact, the oldest rock identified on Earth thus far – four to five billion years old – was found on the Canadian Shield.

The last trees are far south of us. Where we are, we're lucky if a dwarfed birch or a little meadow bush provides a bit of shade. And that is incredibly rare. In contrast to the insects. What a plague! I come to the Northwest Territories with good intentions, equipped with all-natural bug spray and mummified in "bug shirts" and long-sleeved, thin jackets with a hood and face net. But the manufacturer has probably never visited the Far North personally. Here, there is only one solution for human beings: DEET, the abbreviation for diethyl-m-toluamide. It was actually developed for the US-American Army and later used during the Vietnam War; obviously, its health risks were not the foremost criterion. "Over my dead body will I use that stuff!" And two days later, "Give me that spray, will you?" Carefully I spray it over my bug shirt. I am horrified. But it helps just a little bit. Everyone is the same to the mosquitoes; Paul and I are not the only ones struggling with this. All the employees of the diamond mine who work in the open air are also covered from head to foot. And the animal world suffers too: I observe individual caribou that seem to go completely mad, pacing back and forth, snorting and shaking themselves, tossing their heads from side to side and stomping wildly. In her unparalleled documentary film *Being Caribou*, Leanne Allison shows animals burying their noses in the damp moss in desperation, their muzzles festering from the countless insect bites, trying to ease their pain a little. Indeed, the insect scourge is one of the main reasons why many hundreds of thousands of caribou make the long, arduous journey each year from their winter ranges south of the treeline to their calving grounds on the coast of the Arctic Ocean in the Far North. Near the ocean there's a constant, gentle breeze that keeps the mosquito invasion in check; and during the brief summer period, the meadows are lush. Also, there are few big predators here; they remain somewhat farther south but already hungrily await the return of the herds of cows and calves.

This whole arrangement is once again an example of the elaborate interactions in nature. The newborn calves begin to walk within minutes of their birth. After just a few days, they are already accompanying their mothers on the long, dangerous migration to their winter grounds. And very soon, they meet up with the first predators. The Barren Ground grizzlies follow the enormous herds and take the slowest calves. Many more calves die while swimming across the rivers, or are simply separated from their mothers in the crowd and never find them again.

During their trek, eventually the first eskers appear on the horizon. The caribou are entering the land of the wolves at exactly the moment when the wolves have the most important mouths to feed. Their young are now big enough to eat whole chunks of meat by themselves, and preferably lots of them, because the first harbingers of the long, hard winter are already noticeable in early September.

The wolves are once again cleverer than we are. During the day they crouch in their cooler dens for hours, especially to avoid the massive onslaught of bugs. We, on the other hand, are afraid of missing out on something and roast on the heated stone ground beneath us. A feast for the mosquitoes.

A few weeks ago my friend Marco Musiani from the University of Calgary called me. A student, Paul Frame, was looking for someone to assist with his observations of wolf dens in the Barren Grounds. "Yes, yes, of course, I'm in. Tell Paul he can count on me." Then: "What's this all about, anyway?"

"Paul wants to test how wolves behave when their dens are disturbed. First he wants to find suitable dens. Then he'll observe them for three or four days to get familiar with the situation. How many wolves are in the pack, and especially who is who. On the fourth day – at a point when as many wolves as possible are present – he'll approach the den directly and document what happens. For all of that he needs a second person, especially to support him when he approaches the dens. To record everything, the second person will film the whole encounter from a different angle." Wow. Heavy stuff. And exactly the opposite of my other projects, especially the rainforest project. Not only due to the completely different landscape and climate but also because the investigative methods are entirely different. Our code of practice in the rainforest was to be non-invasive, to work without impacting the wolves, without disturbing them. Which can't exactly be said of the design of Paul's study. I stand by my word, nonetheless, because there is a disturbing background to the main question addressed in Paul's line of research. The Far North is being discovered by business. The old, hard Canadian Shield harbours countless valuable natural resources. And humankind has decided that it's about time to use them. In broad explorations, enormous search parties for every possible interest group and industry are sent to the North to locate and retrieve every financially profitable mineral resource.

Paul wants to produce a kind of guide for those working with the search parties that will give them some general information about the wolves. Most important, it is intended to inform them about how they should react if they actually do stumble across wolves and their dens during the course of their work "out there." The results of his current study will form the basis of his recommendations. Still, wouldn't it be possible to find out in a different way, without disturbing the animals? Oh, well. The approach has the blessings of the most famous wolf researcher of them all, Dr. David Mech. Paul is his student.

The Far North has always fascinated me, and the opportunity to observe wolves without the obstacles of trees between us is, of course, the dream of any wolf researcher. And actually of any human being. Even people who don't like wolves want to see and observe them. I recognize what a privilege this is. With mixed

feelings, I fly to Edmonton, the capital of Alberta and the gateway to the North. There I catch a Greyhound bus, the legendary
transportation of all backpackers in North America. At the border
to the Northwest Territories the bus stops in a small town. When
we exit, the mosquitoes devour us for the first time. We board a
new bus, a Grey Goose, fitting for the North. For hours the driver
chauffeurs us along the highway that cuts through the dense boreal forest. Here and there the wall of dark green evergreens opens,
and I can see the reddish-yellow bogs of the North. I will curse
them often in the coming weeks: they are the breeding grounds of
the mosquitoes, the endless numbers of mosquitoes. And the bogs
are hard to cross.

But seen from the inside of the bus, everything is still fine.
After a day and a half of Greyhound and Grey Goose, I arrive at
Yellowknife. Dean Cliff picks me up at the bus stop. He is small
and powerful, his face weathered. Dean brings me to his house.
For several years he has been the wildlife specialist for the government of the Northwest Territories. He is a nice man, and one
with an incredible amount of experience. Paul has already been
under way for more than two months and had another assistant
until recently. I am supposed to replace her for the next few weeks.
The project is supported not only by the government but also by
Canada's first and, at the time, only diamond mine, the Ekati. To
set up the mine, its owner, the Anglo-Australian mineral group
BHP Billiton Ltd., had to go through the most stringent environmental compatibility process in the history of Canada. Which unfortunately doesn't necessarily mean all that much in this country.

NOT ALL THAT GLITTERS IS GOLD
SUMMER 2002

Paul is waiting for me at the mine. Along with some miners flying back to their workplace after their time off, I'm sitting in a big
plane that flies especially for Ekati. I gain wonderful impressions
of the landscape below me: soon after takeoff the forest disperses
into small stands of trees, the areas of moss and bogs become

larger, and then the stark, massive ridges of stone assert themselves. The surface of the lakes between them increases. Then I first see thin, parallel stripes, hundreds of them, no, thousands. At first I can't figure out what they are, but then I understand: caribou trails! Countless. So clearly etched that I can see them from the plane. Over millennia the animals have pressed their mark into the landscape.

Caribou have an enormous impact on the North. They are the pulse of the land, and directly or indirectly all life depends on the tide of them showing up, passing by and disappearing again. They are anticipated, hunted and made use of, then released again and again into the plains of the Arctic coasts, where they reproduce. The flow of nutrients they traditionally activate is gigantic. Around the Ekati mine is the Bathurst herd. In 2006 its population was estimated to be 128,000 animals. By 2009 only 32,000 head were counted.[3] The Aboriginal people of the area point to sport hunters as the cause of this decimation; they in turn point to rapid industrial development of mining and the expansion of the road network. The animals experience additional pressure in those regions where they traditionally give birth to their calves, around Bathurst Inlet, where a large harbour is planned for the anticipated oil tankers and material transport for the development of the last true wilderness regions in North America. In the winter of 2010–2011, for the first time, the famous Northwest Passage was free of ice, which led to jubilation on the part of industry but is a cause of great concern for those involved in worldwide environmental protection. An ice-free passage would allow international freight-ship traffic to finally rush in to make use of a much shorter and politically much more secure shipping route through the Arctic Ocean, not to mention the savings realized by circumventing the Panama Canal. The international race to take possession of the North be-

3 CBC News, "Bathurst Caribou Plan to Help Preserve Herd," October 11, 2010, accessed August 1, 2015, www.cbc.ca/news/canada/north/story/2010/10/11/nwt-bathurst-caribou-wekeezhii-report.html.

gan at the same time. Russians, Americans, Danish and Canadians assess the wilderness, each in hopes of snatching up the biggest piece with the most – and most valuable – mineral resources. Diamonds, rare earth metals for our modern communications technology, and oil. Lots of oil. The results of scientific projects are supposed to provide each government with convincing data to support their legal claims. Each country hopes that, based on the results of geological research related to plate tectonics, the mineral-rich regions will fall under their dominion. Finally, the North can be exploited! Thank you, climate change. Development plans are sprouting like mushrooms. Until recently, the Indigenous peoples of the Canadian North were the guardians of nature. Like all North American First Nations, the lifestyle and culture of the Cree and the Dene were intimately interconnected with their environment. Related, even. Now they are hired by the new industries, for good wages. They work in the diamond pits or build roads. And when that happens, their resistance to the destruction erodes. I am dismayed. In spite of all the environmental protection measures, in the long run, what gets left in the dust is the Far North's extremely fragile ecosystem. Due to the harsh climate, both plants and animals grow extremely slowly. Regeneration takes centuries. Today we know: the pristine North has an expiration date. Until now it has been protected from human exploitation. The barren rock didn't permit cultivation of food; the long winters were too hard on people; the mosquitoes in summer were too irritating. Today, the wilderness is transected by roads that bring construction materials and people into what was once untouched.

I press my nose harder against the window of the plane, not wanting to miss a single caribou trail – there are millions of them. Astonishing how an animal's persistence develops such power that it leaves its traces even on hard rock. I wonder how much longer it will be able to write its story in the bedrock. Without being aware of it, I experience my first "tundra time" up here in the airplane.

At that moment, the first buildings of the diamond-processing facilities appear on the horizon. Like a space station, they stand there like something from a utopian, or dystopian, world. They actually are another world, completely different from the one I have been flying over for the past two hours. The big, angular buildings are all connected to each other by tunnels. There are wide streets everywhere. And two enormous black holes: the pits. Like toys, machines, trucks and cranes move across ramps and storage depots. Immediately I'm aware: not many people get to see this. This is the entrance to hell on Earth.

We land and the workers stream out of the plane. For many of them this is routine, but some are new. They follow the cry of the modern "gold rush" to make a lot of money quickly here. At the first entrance to the main building, however, we are all the same: each of us is thoroughly scanned to make sure nothing illicit enters the camp. The entire establishment is drug-free and there isn't any alcohol either. The litre of whisky I wanted to bring to Paul is disposed of before my eyes. What a shame. On many a cold night in the weeks ahead, I would think longingly of the warming contents of that bottle.

And here comes Paul walking toward me. We've never seen each other before. He is tall and skinny; the past two and a half months have left their mark. It's the end of July and Paul has the period of the midnight sun behind him. The lack of sleep and many hundreds of miles of exploration are written on his face.

We greet each other and Paul gives me a little introduction. In the arrival hall is a glass display case. Inside it a mound of diamonds lies on blue silk. That's the quantity that is mined every day. It's a lot of stones. I learn that the Ekati gems are of especially good quality. A little polar bear is a sign of origin that accompanies every single stone that leaves the mine. Today Ekati diamonds represent 4 per cent of the world's annual production, 4.5 million carats of raw diamonds per year.

Then Paul tries to catch up on his sleep a little, and I get an official tour of the complex. Everything you would never expect to find in such an isolated region is here: a 24-hour self-service buffet, a fitness studio with the most modern equipment I've ever seen, squash and tennis courts, a library, swimming pools, movie theatres. People who work here have a lot of entertainment options, to prevent them from succumbing to cabin fever and coming up with stupid ideas. Lots of distractions to drown out longings. Lots of First Nations people work in the Ekati mine. People who lived on the land and off the land now still live – ironically – off the land but not on it. Everything takes place within the interconnected buildings. Artificial light, artificial air. Shift work around the clock. There's no distinction between day and night. The natural rhythm of the people living inside is completely extinguished. Their senses are befuddled. There are a lot of rules. Otherwise, all of this wouldn't work. One of them is: no going outside. There is a "recreation loop" of just about 3 kilometres that circles the building, but ever since a grizzly was spotted nearby, it has been off limits and won't be opened again this year.

"Paul, when can we finally fly out into the country?"

"There's a helicopter free tomorrow morning." I feel like I've been in this artificial universe for days already. I just want to take one breath of fresh air. The window in my room doesn't open. None of the windows can be opened, because someone could smuggle diamonds out. The sole point of access to the world is through the strictly guarded arrival and departure hall that leads to the plane. Only in winter, for three months of the year, does the almost 500-kilometre-long ice road over the frozen lakes and swamps provide land access to Ekati. Within a few weeks of it freezing, big trucks come, transporting to the mine all the materials needed for the entire year.

I pass the time playing squash with an employee I meet in the lounge. He also dreams of making a quick buck. Bizarre: I had never played squash before and have never played since, only here in this golden cage of civilization in the middle of a beautiful wilderness. In addition to the high standards of environmental protection, the mine owners also have to fulfill a lot of social obligations. The Aboriginal workers receive literacy training, for example.

In the hallway a smartly dressed woman approaches me. "Hello,

Gudrun. I'm Karin, I work here as a teacher. I heard that you're here for a little while. I was born in Germany and am always happy to have a chance to speak German again." Karin tells me that she was hired by the Ekati mine specifically to teach employees to read and write what they need in their workplace. When an employee can read "Warning – danger of lethal electrical shock," it's a big advantage.

An employee from the Dene Nation says he looks forward to going home so much now because he can read his kids a bedtime story. Education is something the people can really use. In this case, however, the Dene Nation are paying a high price for it, namely the loss of their pristine nature and, with it, their roots and their identity.

Similar thoughts come to me when I sit in on a lecture about the company's environmental protection measures. Participation is mandatory for all new employees. I learn that incredibly strict environmental requirements are enforced throughout the operation. There is no plastic packaging anywhere on the compound; the quality of the air and water of the nearby lakes is constantly analyzed. Some of the Dene hunters' traditional knowledge is integrated into environmental management when piles of stone are placed so that caribou are directed away from roads and construction sites. If a caribou still loses its way and wanders into the compound, all traffic at the entrances to construction sites is immediately stopped. I listen to the talk with mixed feelings. Certainly, all these measures are great, but they would not be necessary in the first place if there were no mines. In the meantime, there are six diamond mines in Canada and more are being planned.

Out in the countryside we don't yet notice any of this. It is intensely hot and we are still waiting for some sign of life at the den. On the first day, I could barely tolerate just sitting. Doing absolutely nothing. The time drags. Nothing happens. Everything is calm. Just the constant buzz of insects around me. Still nothing. *My gosh, is this land barren.* Gravel, rocks, little shrubs, a few scattered cushion plants. The air is astonishingly clear. Because of the low humidity, you can see very far; it's hard to estimate exactly how far. There are no reference points in the distance, and I don't have any experience judging distances in such crystal-clear surroundings. No tree to serve as a comparison, nothing. *Man, is this boring!* I furrow my brow in frustration and look over at Paul. At the moment he is scanning the empty horizon with his binoculars, again. Then he wipes the sweat and the pestering mosquitoes from his face. I begin to look into the distance, which blends into the horizon. Somewhere out there, the sky meets Earth. There is no separation anymore. And then it seems as if the sky slowly drapes itself over the rocky landscape. Unspectacular but constant, it sends its envoys. There, something starts to twitter; here, a little bird swings on a delicate branch; over there, an Arctic hare darts from bush to bush; and next to me, humble cushion plants are in bloom. Muskox hairs caught on twigs wave in the breeze, and ahead of me, I recognize the femur of a caribou, bleached from the sun. An Arctic skua rises steeply, then dives onto a ground-breeding bird. My surroundings are teeming with life and full of things just waiting to be discovered. They tell me their stories, and in fine, subtle hints, generously whisper the mysteries of the tundra to me. Did they really just appear? Or were they always there and I just never noticed them, never devoted my full attention to them? Did I overlook them? The next hours I continue to just sit there, but I am no longer waiting; I observe, learn, am occupied and amazed. At some point Paul nudges me.

"Gudrun, look! A wolf is coming out of the den!"

"Oh, right, the wolves … that's why we're here."

I never tire of just watching them. Even if the two adult wolves aren't really doing much of anything. There they stand. Thick bunches of fur still hang from their very pale, almost-white coats. No sooner have they lost their thick, long winter coat than they have to slowly start preparing themselves for the next cold season, like so many tundra inhabitants. Some avoid the cold in a different way: they fly away from it or they migrate. Like the herds of caribou that move to the protective forests to the South in August.

We expect the herds to move through in the next few days. These animals are a huge factor in the economy of the region. The local Aboriginal peoples traditionally use every bit of the caribou, from the meat to the tendons, the warm fur to the bones and antlers. And then there are numerous hunters from around the world who stalk the animals for the sake of a trophy each year. Both sexes bear the typical antlers, but, like everywhere, the sport hunters find the bigger the better.

While the migration follows traditional routes each year, there are an incredible number of possible routes. The many factors that determine which path the herds take and when remain their secret. And that remains so in spite of the fact that for years now several individuals in each herd have been wearing satellite radio collars; thanks to them, government wildlife biologists can follow the migrations on computer screens from their offices in Yellowknife.

The wolves have no high-tech devices to locate their prey. Still, we notice they are becoming more active and staying away from the den longer. They set off to hunt at almost the exact same time every evening; it's a routine process. The female stands up first, stretches, and slowly walks over to her partner. Then they greet each other with wagging tails and lick each other. She determines which direction they head, and he is always fine with that. He ambles along behind her. As I follow them with the binoculars, they are always swallowed up by the land and, after a while, are spit out again in a different spot: the lack of dimensionality makes it very difficult to recognize surface features; little knolls or ditches melt into the land completely. The wolves disappear from sight again and again.

The next morning, we are back at our observation posts when the male wolf returns to the den. The female seems to have come home earlier. As he approaches, we can see he is carrying a caribou leg in his mouth. He is boisterously greeted and surrounded by his family. It's not only the other wolves that are thrilled; we are also on high alert. Caribou! The wolf actually managed to locate, hunt and kill a caribou in this endless expanse, to then schlep it back to his family piece by piece. What an incredible accomplishment by the head of the family! We don't yet know anything about the caribou in our surroundings, even though Paul is in contact with Dean in Yellowknife via satellite phone daily. From a technical perspective, we are informed about where the herd should be. But the keen senses of the old wolf show us the reality.

When we crawl sleepily out of our tent in the morning a few days later, there is something in the air. Today something is different than usual. I look around me. Behind the rise just a few hundred metres away from our tent, I see them: new and old, freshly churned-up paths, hoof prints big and small, coming from the north. The caribou must have rushed past our camping spot and disappeared toward the south again. On the little branches of the dwarf shrubs hang bunches of hair, and the scent of fresh droppings fills the morning air. There is now a slight hint of urgency in this otherwise peaceful and calm morning. They moved through during the night, while we slept deeply and dreamed of them. I'm a little disappointed to have missed this spectacle, to be honest, but soon I recall the wolf's catch a few days ago. And I'm happy for the wolf family that they have such an abundance of food, for a short time at least. During the day we do see a few individual caribou.

We are lucky: no sooner has the Ekati helicopter brought us safely to the mine complex than a storm breaks out that keeps us imprisoned there for three days. Just a little bit later and the helicopter wouldn't have been able to evacuate us anymore. This time I am grateful for this oasis of civilization. It's one thing to ride out the powerful storm in here, but I constantly think about the wolves and especially the young caribou calves that have to pass this first test of their endurance out in the elements.

When the weather finally improves, we fly out into the backcountry to another wolf's lair. And once again we put up our tents about 3 kilometres away from the den, look for an observation point – hidden from the wolves – about a kilometre from it, for three days record as many details as possible of the wolves' everyday behaviour at the site, and on the third or fourth day execute the "disrupt the wolf pack at their den" campaign. What will stay with me forever is how deeply the reactions of all the wolves at all the dens shame me. These animals, viewed by many uninformed people as dangerous beasts, always want just one thing: to bring their young to safety and escape from the threat that is coming right at them on two legs. Paul stands erect and moves quickly. The wolves seem to be completely beside themselves, but it quickly becomes clear why there is a certain role for each animal within the pack. The lead male wolf runs toward Paul barking and always remains between him and the family, keeping a respectful distance. This is his desperate attempt to keep the intruder from coming any closer to his nursery. But Paul continues without wavering. In the meantime, the mother and other adult wolves have rounded up the pups and fled with them. Finally, the father, sometimes supported by a second high-ranking wolf, depending on the size of the pack, also leaves the scene and cedes the den to Paul. Again and again this is how the test plays out, or very similarly. Distraught, I ponder why it is that animals that boldly take on grizzly bears or can kill wildly thrashing prey that weighs several hundred kilograms with a single bite – why would they flee from us humans so helplessly and without any defence at all? What must they have been through with our species that they are so afraid of us? It is mortifying and shameful, just shameful. Here in the still expanses of the North, the wolf turns its reputation as a ravenous killer completely on its head. I want to transport this scene farther south with me, somehow. There, where people have no conception of what wolves truly are.

Events at the very last wolf's den demonstrate clearly that the wolf can behave differently. Here, instead of disturbing the den as a human, Paul wants to sneak up close to them and then – hidden behind a rock – howl like an intruding wolf.

What happens next is beyond our expectations. Paul hides himself behind a big boulder. He howls very well and the wolves fall for his imitation completely. Again the alpha male and a second adult wolf dart directly toward the source of the howling, but this time they don't stop and stand at a certain distance. Quite the opposite: they move faster and faster, their bounds become longer and higher, their hackles bristle, and their ears and lips indicate they're on the attack. The pair of them run with determination toward the boulder behind which Paul is still keeping hidden. I observe all of this from my hideout, which is at a right angle to the direction the wolves are running. "Paul! Hey, these two are serious. Do something! Show yourself to them before they get to the boulder!" I scream into the walkie-talkie. And Paul jumps out from behind his rock. In the same moment, the wolves see him. One manages the incredible feat of doing an about face mid-jump and turning away. The other comes to an immediate halt. Both look like something out of a bad cartoon. The first wolf runs back, barking, and positions himself between his alarmed family and Paul; the second scales a cliff with a flat ledge, where he howls for several minutes.

The next day, the den has been abandoned. We look for the wolf family. They can't be too far away; the pups are still not big enough to make long treks. Suddenly we notice something big and dark on the small hill. It's moving. "Quick, the binoculars!" We both cry almost simultaneously, "A grizzly!" A big Barren Ground grizzly bear is standing on the crest. It seems to be eating something. Yes, there's a dead caribou lying there. I continue to observe the bear while Paul frantically unpacks his video camera. Then a white wolf appears at the foot of the hill, stops for a moment, then moves confidently toward the big bear. Is he crazy, interfering with a grizzly at its kill all by himself? I press the binoculars closer to my face. The wolf has reached the bear. Suddenly he jumps at the grizzly and bites it in the left hind leg. The bear whirls around and makes a quick lunge at the wolf. The wolf neatly evades it, moves a few steps farther away and lies down right near the bear. With its legs outstretched, not ready to jump, not even on alert. The scene doesn't change for a while now; the bear continues to feed and the wolf seems to accept it patiently. When the bear has had its fill, it disappears behind the hill. The wolf stands up, goes over to what's left of the carcass, pulls on it a little and then walks off in the direction he came from.

Now we notice life in the small basin to which the wolf retreats: one, two, three wolves and several small, dark pups are there. These are our "lost wolves." And they have a new rendezvous site. A rendezvous site is where the wolf pups are watched by their "babysitters" and raised after they leave their dens, and where the rest of the pack gathers during the summer months. The father wolf probably wanted to try to bring his family some of the caribou and was willing to risk a confrontation with the bear. It doesn't seem like he took it too seriously. Both the wolf and the bear were a bit half-hearted when you consider how rare (and thus valuable) food is in this region. I expect more intense conflicts.

The mystery is solved two days later. The wolf family has moved again and the bear has followed them. It looks very much like the bear is a familiar acquaintance of this pack and that this wasn't the first time the bear has helped itself to the wolves' catch. The bear lets the wolves do the dirty work of hunting and killing the caribou, and then shows up to claim the fresh delicacy. The wolves seem to accept this arrangement. In exchange, the grizzly leaves the pack, and especially its pups, in peace. These are the little trade-offs that take place in the Barren Grounds.

A SPECIAL VISITOR
SUMMER 2002

Slowly Alan guides his seaplane in its descent. Another lake appears on the horizon – one of millions – but one of the few with a name: Aylmer Lake. Alan owns Aylmer Lake Lodge on the northeastern shore. From the air I see the simple, small cabins and the main building. They are nestled along a barren little spit of land that extends into the lake. Elegantly, Alan circles his Cessna above the lodge. We land on the glass-clear water and motor to the dock. Rick, Alan's younger son, jumps onto the plane's pontoons with a thick rope in his hand and ties it to the dock with practised motions. Slowly, we peel ourselves out of the match-box-sized plane, Alan, Paul, and I. We also have Alan's shopping from Yellowknife and our mountain of gear with us. The groceries have to sustain the entire operations of the lodge for the next two weeks. That's the next time Alan will fly to the capital city again, a flight of more than two hours. At the moment, there are a couple of fishermen and caribou hunters staying here. In addition to his two sons, Alan has hired Henry Basil, of the Dene First Nation, as a guide for his hunting guests. These guys grew up on the land and know the caribou migration routes and the best fishing spots like the backs of their hands. They advertise "world-class fishing for lake trout, arctic grayling and northern pike," and rightly so. The overweight, loud US-Americans at the next table are planning their caribou hunt for the next day. And bits of their fishing jargon drift over to us. Paul, himself an enthusiastic angler, perks up his ears when he hears the current numbers: lake trout weighing about 18 kilograms.

That afternoon we also fish for a little while, catch and release only. So we catch fish, measure them and toss them back in the water. I watch Paul – he is good. And I ask myself why people tear the fishes' mouth and damage the protective layer of slime on their scales, just to capture the moment by taking a photo with them.

Kathy, Alan's wife, is a good cook. Alan has lots of fascinating stories to tell and is a big fan of wolves. He has made many wolf-scouting tours with his little plane, just for his own pleasure. He is a big help in deciding where we will spend the next few days. "I think you two should go to the southwest end of the lake. On my last flight I saw a couple of wolves running along the esker. They must have a den there." We gratefully accept his offer and the next morning make an exploratory flight. Aylmer Lake is large, almost 60 kilometres long and more than 25 kilometres wide. As we fly over the esker, two wolves walk diagonally across its sandy surface and disappear behind the peak. Alan turns around.

Back at the lodge, we take over a motorboat and set off on the lake toward the esker we just saw. Motivated by the sighting, we set up our camp right at the stunningly beautiful lakeshore. The yellow sand beach slowly disappears into the lake, which, due to its size, behaves more like an ocean and sends waves toward the beach in regular, gentle beats. The sound of longing. The vivid colours of the North intensify toward evening, when we finally sit at a campfire. With pleasure we dig into the fresh food that Kathy quickly slipped in among our things. Fresh food like fruit or vegetables, cheese or cold cuts are a luxury. In addition to their short shelf life, they also have a major disadvantage: they provide few calories but take a lot of space. What we need is exactly the opposite because each of us has only one relatively small, black, cylinder-shaped box made of thick plastic to contain our entire food ration for about a week. These boxes are the only objects in our camp that are bear-safe. The lid of the box shuts seamlessly at the edge and can only be opened with a coin or something similar – and then with difficulty. The entire box has no gripping surface and likes to roll away. Perfect design – even a rather imaginative grizzly can't break into it. But the boxes are small. That's why Paul and I went out in the boat briefly to augment our evening meal: a freshly caught fish coated in Kathy's famous breading mix is in a completely different league than three-minute instant pasta. It takes longer than we expected to land the right fish. Not because they weren't biting but because the many fish we caught were too big for just the two of us. And we wanted neither to waste leftover fish nor to invite bears into our camp with it.

Now we are sitting on the shore of the lake, well satisfied, each with a cup of coffee for dessert – there always has to be room for that in the bear box. Contemplatively, I look over at Paul. His last sentence stuck in my conscience: "The fish we had for dinner must have been 30 years old." Thirty? Thirty years? And we eat it in just a few minutes? Yes, time takes on other dimensions here. Everything moves more slowly; the long winter has a grip on the land for at least eight months and stops all growth. The oldest stones in the world don't easily let themselves be eroded by the tentatively growing plants and the acidity of their roots.

Everything that lives and breathes here is extremely precious. The beauty lies in the barrenness.

The next morning we set off in search of the esker and the den we presume is there. Paul saved the coordinates in his GPS when we circled above it yesterday. We are moving toward wolves. When we cross a small plateau, we stumble across a piece of rusting iron. Where did that come from? Little things you wouldn't even notice at home are a big deal here and take on significance. I bend down and pull on the metal, overgrown with plants: it's a foothold trap. Now we look more closely under the meagre growth: there are more of them! With our bare hands we uncover one after the other. In the end there are almost 30. All of them are old and rusted and no longer have chains. Thank heavens they're not set anymore, but they are still fully functional. "V" for Victoria Falls is emblazoned on the round pan. The classic trap from the bloody period of fur trapping. Paul's eyes begin to shine. "I'm taking these home with me! They're still good enough for foxes. And a historical treasure." Rusty junk, I think, taking one for myself as a reminder of the bloody butchering conducted by the first white people in the North 150 years ago.

We want to bring them to our camp on our way back. Nearby, we find remnants of an old cabin. For a long time, trapping and the fur trade were the only reasons Europeans ventured into the North. But for a few decades they were richly rewarded for their trials and tribulations: the pelts of Arctic foxes and wolves are especially dense and brought good prices on the European fashion market. Rotten boards and rusty iron tell the story even today. As we continue to hike, we discover wooden stakes with markings in neon colours – claim stakes. Someone has already snatched up this land. Probably an international mining company that hopes to find, or has already found, something valuable deep underneath the tundra mosses and lichens. If the hunt used to be for resources that the land yielded, like furs and meat, today the hunt is for things the land itself consists of. What both kinds of hunters share in common is that, ironically, they are looking for riches in a landscape dominated by scarcity. It's bizarre, but they do hit pay dirt here. And can become rich. But the slow pace and the beauty of the land are never revealed to them.

On our way back we gather as many traps as we can stuff into our backpacks. When we get to camp, Paul calls Dean in Yellowknife via satellite phone. He tells him about our successful search for the wolf's den first, and then about all the traps we found. "Wow, that's fantastic! I hope you got the exact UTM coordinates of the site. That's a historical find. Leave everything exactly the way you found it. Fabulous!" Dean is enthusiastic. Paul and I look at each other, then at the pile of traps on the ground next to us. The next morning, grumbling, we schlep them all back to the exact places where they've been rusting away for several decades. I think Paul is really sad that he can't try out the traps in Minnesota. But as non-Canadians, we follow the Canadian regulations to the letter, even when they are sometimes mystifying to us.

As we do at every den, we observe the wolf family's activities – or lack of activity, is more like it. During the day, they leave us entirely to the mosquitoes, but in the morning and evening hours, the animals are lively. In this pack there seem to be two females with pups. This is not typical, because usually only one female raises a litter, the leading female of the pack. But in the North, multiple litters are probably a compensation strategy for the especially high mortality rate of pups at this latitude.

It's another beautiful morning. The air is already cool in mid-September, and especially at this time of year the night quickly reclaims the hours of daylight loaned to the summer. Almost ten minutes every day, more than an entire hour of additional darkness each week.

The morning sun is just rising above the lake. I want to go down to the water to wash. That's odd, where is our cooking tent? We always set it up a few hundred metres away from our sleeping tent. As I come closer, a cold shiver runs down my back. It's totally flattened, side flaps are torn, blood on the mangled metal stakes: we have had a visitor during the night. A grizzly bear completely dismantled our cooking tent, while we slept right nearby, not suspecting a thing. Its enormous paw prints in the sand trace the trail of devastation. Instinctively I turn around and look in every direction, although I know it's no longer close by. But what will happen in the coming night? Has the bear become eager for more, or did it give up on our location because it wasn't rewarded with food?

Paul is completely distraught about the bear visit and blames us both for not being careful enough with our food; I think the bear was just able to catch the scent of food on the walls of the tent with its incredibly sensitive nose. Both of our bear boxes lie exactly where we stashed them, untouched. Paul is torn; we still have to spend two nights here to complete the sequence of the project. He calls Dean.

"Where exactly did you put up the mess tent?" Grizzlies don't scare Dean so easily.

"On the sand right near the shore of the lake."

"Well, that makes sense. Grizzlies like to roam along the beach. Your tent was probably just in the way, and the bear removed it, in its own special way."

Okay, that makes sense, I think to myself. Except for the fact that we might have a raving Barrens grizzly bear as a neighbour in the coming night, everything is fine.

On our way to the wolf den, we see the bear. It likes this area. Good for the bear. But the next evening, I keep my bear spray especially close at hand, and my pocket knife next to my head. Sleep is out of the question. Paul even has his gun with him. The night remains calm, and we never see the grizzly bear again. And to be honest, we didn't miss it, either.

ATTITUDES
SUMMER 2002

Paul stands next to me, tall and haggard. He has just taken his gun from his shoulder and loaded it. I stare at him in disbelief. *Why is that necessary?* I think, turning my gaze back to the silhouette of the Barren Ground grizzly bear that's casually wandering across the tundra. It must be 500 metres away. We are standing west of the bear on a nondescript hill. The wind is coming from the west. I assume the bear knows we're here, but it stays on its original course, which runs parallel to the direction we are heading. For me, this is a sign that everything is okay for now. I soak in the peaceful sight of the beautiful animal moving easily through this empty landscape. At some point, it disappears between the boulders. Paul remains on high alert and ready to shoot the entire time. The two of us are standing side by side, are in the same situation, see the same thing. And yet our reactions are so different, because we have had completely different experiences. Paul is a biologist but also a trapper and hunter. He lives in Minnesota, where there are countless black bears but no grizzlies. I have just come from Heiltsuk Territory, and their overall attitude, full of respect for all living things, is at the forefront of my stash of memories. My US-American friend Carol said something that will stick with me for the rest of my life. "Gudrun, always think: stress is not the event, it is only *your* reaction." In other words, I often can't influence the event, but my reaction to it is a different story. I can consciously guide my response.

I feel that Paul's reaction could perhaps trigger something unnecessary. What it definitely provoked was a somewhat heated discussion about gun ownership and use. Paul's background for his position is the Second Amendment of the United States Constitution, which was adopted in 1791 as part of the Bill of Rights and ratified by 11 states. It reads: "A well regulated Militia, being necessary to the security of a free State, the right of the people to keep and bear Arms, shall not be infringed."[4] This amendment continues to be a key component of many US-Americans' understanding of themselves. The right to own and use a gun is something they take for granted.

I just look at Paul wordlessly as he builds a case based on exactly

4 See "Amendment II," accessed July 2, 2015, www.senate.gov/civics/constitution_item/constitution.htm#amdt_2_(1791).

this legal principle. As he explains his position, the magnitude of the effect this right has on social interaction, not only throughout his society but also that of our entire world, slowly begins to dawn on me. I cannot get used to the idea of taking potential danger into consideration every time people interact with each other.

A few days after the first grizzly sighting, it's my birthday. My 30th. When I was younger, so many of my dreams for the future began with, "When I'm 30, I'll be … I'll know … I'll…" And? I own nothing (in terms of material goods), and what do I really know about anything? This matter-of-fact assessment makes me sad. For a few moments I even doubt if researching wolves and following their tracks, alone, are really fulfilling.

A snowstorm keeps Paul and me at the Aylmer Lake Lodge for two days. When the storm finally eases, I give myself the gift of a walk across the tundra. Everything is bathed in cloudy grey; the infinite sky hangs deep over the flat terrain. Plumes of mist from the lake drift close to the rocky ground, mystically. Everything is so peaceful. Nothing is moving. The weather is perfect for moping, and so I really wallow in my misery. I think about big parties to celebrate 30th birthdays, about lots of smiling and celebrating friends, about the things I had hoped to achieve, about the words "We love you. We're so happy you're here!" Everything is so far away, so unreal for me right now. I look into the grey nothingness ahead of me. And then suddenly there's movement in the dismal scenery; I notice something in the distance coming toward me. Dark, four legs. I stand still, crouch down and wait. It continues to come closer. Undeterred and unconcerned, a wolverine lopes in my direction. Then it slows down, coming to a walk a few metres away from me, and looks at me with its big, dark eyes. I watch it. If I stretched out my hand right now, I could touch it. The animal lifts its nose then walks right past me, picking up its pace, and disappears again into the fog at a wolverine gallop. I stay there for a few more minutes – unbelievable. And I smile. All self-doubt is forgotten. At all the birthday parties in the world, who has ever had a wolverine come to congratulate them? I am thrilled. I only become aware of the real significance later, when I give a report of my encounter back at the lodge. The owner and the majority of the guests go wild: "Gudrun, that's totally crazy! We've never heard of anything like it. My God, it could have killed you!"

Wolverines are the largest members of the weasel family. There are lots of dreadful legends told about them because, like all weasels, they are very bold for their size – 20 to 30 kilograms and up to 1.3 metres long – and can be aggressive. A single wolverine can even take down a caribou that weighs ten times as much as it does. Its technique is to jump onto the back of its prey and bite it on the neck. A wolverine won't even refrain from fighting a bear to take its food. In German, they are called *Vielfrass*, derived from the Nordic term *Fjellfräs*, which means something like mountain cat. The English word "wolverine" is related to "wolf."

Now I'm smiling again. "No, I don't think it would have…"

THE ETERNAL DANCE OF THE HUNTERS AND THE HUNTED
LATE SUMMER 2002

"Gudrun, while the others are just observing the muskox, look all around you, because the wolves are sure to be nearby." Henry would know. He is a part of the land. His ancestors have lived on and from the land for millennia. Like all people who spend a lot of time out in nature, he has developed a fine sense for what's going on around him. Henry acknowledges the meaning and significance of what is happening. And so a deep connection and intimate understanding has developed. It is always wonderful to spend time with such people. Your own life is intensified and enriched, and I am deeply content.

So I look to the south, and at that very moment I see a white wolf and a black wolf trotting toward the muskox herd. I nod at Henry with appreciation and gratitude. He sits next to me with his long, black hair in two braids held together with caribou-leather bands. He gave me two pair of these bands, as well: brown for the summer and white for the winter. Then we went outside the lodge, and in a small ceremony he showed me the right way to plait a braid and to pray to the Great Spirit as you do it. "Always braid from the outside to the inside. That's important. And wrap the leather band around the end four times, once for each of the four directions," Henry explained. Now I have a better understanding of the importance of long hair for all First Nations. And the psychic pain the white missionaries must have inflicted on young First Nations children when they cut off their long hair the moment they entered the government-mandated residential schools they were forced to attend.

Again and again I encounter the aftermath of these governmental–missionary institutions. Until the 1960s they systematically and brutally tried to turn Aboriginal peoples into white people, obliterating their identity, culture, language, stories, knowledge and ways of life. The goal was to destroy them as what they were and to impose the Western system of values on them. The children were torn from their villages and put in boarding schools far away from their families. They were not allowed to speak their languages, had to wear uniforms, and were forced to adopt the lifestyle of the white people. The ancient chain of oral transmission of all traditions from the Elders to their children and youth was successfully interrupted. Successful? When the young people were released from their schools, they were in a spiritual and emotional no man's land, and they were homeless. They didn't understand their parents anymore, but they weren't orphans either. Striving to acquire possessions, saving and planning for the future – the whole egocentric worldview of the West – remained foreign to them, in spite of the educators' extreme efforts. The federal residential schools produced generations of confused, misunderstood and disoriented people, traumatized by violence and abuse. The purpose of the institutions was "to kill the Indian in the child." The last school of this kind in Canada wasn't closed until 1996.[5]

5 Gordon Indian Residential School, near Punnichy, Saskatchewan. See "Residential Church School Scandal," *Maclean's*, June 26, 2000, accessed August 2, 2015, www.thecanadianencyclopedia.ca/en/article/residential-church-school-scandal/.

On June 11, 2008, after years of lawsuits by victims and legal proceedings related to restitution payments, Prime Minister Stephen Harper made an official apology on behalf of the government for the policy of assimilation of the First Nations that had been implemented by the Canadian government.[6] Harper apologized not only for the abuse that took place in the schools but also for their very existence. The speech took place before a delegation of Canadian First Nations peoples and was broadcast live by the CBC television network.

At the time, I happen to be in Bella Bella, centre of the Heiltsuk First Nation, and experience the broadcast as one of two white people in the packed auditorium of the community centre along with many survivors of the residential schools. The situation is moving. But I am truly struck by the reactions of the people gathered after the speech. For the First Nations of North America, words have an immense import. They are therefore used sparingly. They may not talk much, but what they say is carefully considered and also carefully listened to. Harper's speech has ended. After a longer silence in the room, one of the Elders slowly stands up and walks calmly to the podium. In simple and very clear words he tells his story. There is a reverent silence in the auditorium. Then a second person rises, and a third, and so on. The room is filled with aching souls who speak about harrowing experiences. They have had to wait decades for this day. Full of gratitude that they can finally talk about it officially now, they give their deeply buried feelings free rein. The most miraculous thing, though, is that they continually remind and encourage each other not to file suits or seek revenge but to forgive. I can see how difficult it is for them, but they have this ability within them drawn from the greatness of their people, and by banding together they find strength.

6 CBC News, "PM Cites 'Sad Chapter' in Apology for Residential Schools," accessed August 2, 2015, www.cbc.ca/news/canada/pm-cites-sad-chapter-in-apology-for-residential-schools-1.699389.

I feel very uncomfortable in my white skin. But the longer the speeches go on, the more burdens are cast off and a collective relief fills the room. The foundation stone for a new kind of coexistence has officially been laid. The scars will remain forever.

Many First Nations honour the wolf. And with the increasingly intense presence of Western cost-benefit analysis, their fate was not much different than that of the wolf. Both seemed to be unprofitable and unnecessary in the eyes of white people. Anachronous. So many First Nations have historically identified with the fate of the wolf. Both wolves and Indigenous peoples were hunters on the continent for millennia who managed to ensure their own survival without annihilating to complete extinction the population of the animals they preyed on.

The Europeans came and brought new, efficient weapons to the First Nations and easy-to-kill domesticated animals for the wolf. Both had fatal consequences for the traditional hunting methods of the original inhabitants, threw them out of balance. The hunters unexpectedly found themselves in completely new circumstances: all of a sudden the hunt and killing became so much easier. Within a short time, and with little effort and risk, so much more could be caught. The hunters' behaviour wasn't adapted to this situation. And even today, wolves are still getting used to this utterly new circumstance that had never existed before. Unfortunately, some First Nation peoples "sell" their natural heritage to hunting parties or even themselves shoot animals that have become rare, only to sell them on the black market. And the wolves search out the prey that are easiest to catch: domesticated animals.

In the 1990s, at the latest, it became clear that the land was missing something essential without First Nations cultures and without wolves, and so a wave of reparations began to sweep across the continent. In Canada it was the long overdue and longed-for apology for the policies of cultural genocide practised during the preceding decades, and in the United States the reintroduction of wolves in the most famous and oldest national park in the world: Yellowstone, in Wyoming, Montana and Idaho. This reintroduction received decisive support from the local Nez Perce people. They saw in this act a kind of reconciliation of the white people with their people.

Both the First Nations and the wolves are recovering slowly, very slowly, from their shared fate. And at the same time there are limits: in the summer of 2011 the United States removed the wolf from its list of endangered species (then reinstated the protection in the winter of 2015), and many First Nations peoples still live on their reserves today.

Henry smiles modestly. He notices my implied shake of the head. Mystified, I follow the two wolves that he just predicted a moment ago. They only stand still occasionally to turn around and look for the other one. I think I'm in the middle of one of those spectacular hunting scenes in a Discovery Channel production. The muskox herd is still grazing calmly, not suspecting a thing. Together with the group of American wolf watchers led by Dr. Dave Mech, we are sitting on a small rise on a peninsula in Aylmer Lake. The terrain rolls gently, and the slope opposite us is covered with rare, juicy greens that attract the herbivores. The peninsula is only connected to the mainland by a narrow bridge of land. The shaggy muskox have to cross it in order to reach the feeding grounds. And exactly there a small wolf family has established its den. Strategically perfect. The cameras of the American eco-tourists click; they are still focused on the muskox herd. A few of the participants come here every year to have a live experience of wild wolves living freely. They pay a lot of money for it, and their camera equipment is correspondingly expensive. I think to myself how great it is that they pay a bunch of money and I get to see this for free. The weeks I am spending with Paul represent a volunteer opportunity, true, but I don't have any expenses and get to experience things that enrich me forever. A wealth that isn't subject to inflation; just the opposite: the longer I carry the memories of this time in the North with me, the more valuable they become. They help me again and again in the course of my life when I need motivation or am feeling an inner emptiness. Moments like these don't disappear; they defy time, which works toward decay. They are part of a wealth that you can't buy for all the money in the world.

The pair of wolves now comes into view of the paying tourists. Excitedly, the sightseers turn their telescopic lenses toward the wolves. All of them are in suspense. They are all familiar with the famous action film and photo sequence of the white wolves of Ellesmere Island hunting muskox. Through his more than 25 years of observing these wolves in the High Arctic, Dave Mech has risen into the pantheon of wolf research. He is *the* wolf researcher. When I met him in person a few days earlier, an endearing but perhaps a little quirky older man stood before me. He still advances the "old school" of wolf research: he doesn't shy away from invasive methods as long as we can expect to gain new information from them. Debatable. And in complete contrast with the research philosophy of Dr. Paul Paquet, whose work is geared toward providing a scientific basis for the protection of big animals of prey and their habitats with hard facts. And in the process, respect for the sensibilities of animals living in the wild is his first priority. Paul and Dave represent such different perspectives that they have fruitful consequences for the entire field of research. Dave's approach should, however, be phased out.

The wolves separate. The black one remains between us and the herd, while the lighter one disappears to the left behind a crest. A little later it reappears above the ungulates. What is it up to? Will it force the animals toward its partner? We hardly dare to breathe. Will the most archaic of all wilderness scenes play out before our very eyes in the next few minutes? The dance between life and death? The driving force of evolution, the progressive development of survival of the fittest? The black wolf sniffs in the depression between us and the herbivores and so far takes no interest in the herd or in the other wolf. Suddenly it becomes animated: it darts forward, jumps up with its front paws raised, propelling itself with its hind legs and immediately lands again on its front legs. It has caught a mouse. For the next two hours the black wolf does nothing else. It adroitly catches mice. We don't catch another glimpse of the white wolf before we leave.

It is a myth that hunters are continually on the hunt and prey is constantly on the run. In nature both sides have one thing in common: the wise use and conserve their energy. Hunters demonstrate this by observing their potential prey for hours, even days. They want to figure out which animal in the herd is growing weaker and thus offers the greatest chance to obtain food with the least possible risk and loss of energy. And the prey animals are used to living with their predators. In fact, they even want to stand their ground around their enemies, because that demonstrates strength and superiority. And above all, this behaviour also conserves precious energy. Running away every time a familiar enemy is simply in the vicinity makes no sense in terms of energy retention. Prey animals that have experience with their predators have developed a sense for when the situation becomes serious and when they can tolerate a wolf nearby. We were able to observe this again and again in Canada, in different regions and ecosystems with diverse wolf populations and diverse types of prey. The often cited balance in the tumult of nature, however, doesn't exist; it is instead an oscillation around a more or less stable middle. A constant up and down, permanent change, a building up and breaking down. Dynamism is the precondition for life and for all vital functions. We human beings find it difficult when this kind of cycle doesn't go our way or fit with what we imagine. But in our short-sightedness we often deprive nature of this room to vacillate.

In every respect, wild animals demonstrate expedient adaptation strategies. We just need to be prepared to part with our expectations. Today the wolf-watching group and I do not take away spectacular impressions of hunting and killing. But we have learned more about the wolf than we anticipated at first. While we people often make a mountain out of a molehill, the black wolf made mice out of muskox – and still returned to the den with a full belly. It adapted to its circumstances and made the best out of them.

WOLF SPIRIT 9
NOVEMBER 2005

Thirty-two units of radiation coupled with the chemotherapy. Both have to happen within an hour. The chemo looks harmless, a little white tablet like many others, nothing special. But it packs a powerful punch. After the first dose I have to throw up; then my body gradually gets used to the poison, at least temporarily. I set the alarm, because I scheduled all my radiation appointments first thing in the morning. I prefer that; then I have the whole thing behind me sooner and have more freedom to plan my day. I have to take the chemo pill an hour before the radiation. Not on an empty stomach, but I have to be finished eating an hour before taking the chemo. Soon nothing tastes good, and after a few more days I can't tolerate anything at all. The only thing I can still get down is potatoes. Potatoes without anything. Potatoes for breakfast, lunch and dinner. My friends are doubtful, but I stick with it.

In the waiting room for radiation treatments I meet a young woman about my age. She has three children and a brain tumour, stage IV, the most aggressive form and in an inoperable location. Tanja is cheerful and entertaining, extroverted and doesn't complain. Her presence not only helps the waiting fly by, she also reminds me simply by her presence that I don't really have it bad. But she looks fabulous, no swelling of her face due to the strong steroids that we both have to take in high doses to keep the massive swelling in our brains under control following surgery. "Moon face" is the term for it, and it's very descriptive. While my body gets thinner and thinner from the neck down, my face fills out to resemble a full moon. After half of the radiation treatments, I suddenly lose my hair, long at the time, by the handful. Until I hear from my new therapist in Canmore, Christian: "Gudrun, own it. Shave it all off. Wear a black turtleneck and beautiful earrings. You'll look great." I follow his advance and do a little better. I still ask the question and the radiation team says, "We don't know, but you are getting an especially high dose. It could be that your hair will never grow back. But these days there are such natural looking wigs." Once again a setback, again such a challenge, another act of mental power. Now I have my own hair again, and only if you know where to look, you can see an area where the hair is thinner and ever so slightly lighter in colour. And the only thing the moon face left behind was a few more wrinkles. I can live with those, happily. Dr. Sung answered my question about the long-term consequences of the radiation very curtly: "Yes, they will probably intensify, especially your concentration and your ability to memorize will decrease." Unfortunately, she wasn't entirely wrong about that, but when I've forgotten something again I just smile and say, "Well, I do have a hole in my brain."

My life decelerates, especially during the first months on the couch. Nothing else is possible. And during the next two years, my entire life revolves around healing.

Phil writes a detailed plan – typical Phil.

Steps Gudrun must take to get healthy again!

1. DON'T DO MORE THAN TWO *things a day (at most one hour each)*

2. *Say* NO *to visitors and other things that are too much for you.*

3. *Be* PATIENT *with your recovery, especially when you feel* GOOD: *take advantage of that feeling and* HANG ON TO IT – DON'T WASTE IT *on anyone or anything else.*

4. *Gain some* WEIGHT. *Goal: 55 kg*

5. *Always keep your eyes on the horizon.*

Touched

WILD ISLAND

THE WOLF'S MESSAGE
SEPTEMBER 2005

"And? How was it? Finally find something?" Jean Marc stands in a wide stance in his small aluminum boat as he picks up Richard, Simon and me at the end of the little cove. I furtively roll my eyes, and he gets the message even before the two film people open their mouths. The mood is already rather muted; just about three weeks have gone by since Richard and Simon have been on board with us. And we haven't yet gotten a single wolf in front of the camera lens. I'm frustrated because I see little chance for our last few days unless the two-man camera crew quickly changes its approach to getting close to them. Stomping through the forest with big, heavy cameras is no way to film wolves. You have to give yourself and the wolves lots of time for that to happen. Sitting still, hiding yourself and waiting calmly is the magic formula, but for a long time Richard doesn't want to accept that. By the time his professionalism finally triumphs over his restless drive, it's almost too late. The camera team's plane flies back to South Africa in two days. We've just received a radio message that wolf howling has been heard in a meadow near a remote estuary on an outer coast island. Jean Marc immediately changes course and navigates his *Tilsup* into the little cove next to the stream.

It's the middle of the day, and after scrutinizing the meadow with binoculars, it looks like nothing is happening there at the moment. Carefully, I take in our surroundings. The river should be full of salmon at this time of year, but I see only three of them in the water. And there are no signs of wolves having caught salmon along the shore, either. I am disappointed. But it makes sense: where there are no salmon, none can be caught and eaten. Still, I soon find well-worn wolf tracks in the tall grass, then a fresh deer-leg bone, cracked in the wolves' way. Back on the boat, we know it's now or not at all. And we come up with a risky plan: we will stay here. In the next days, Richard and Simon build themselves a small hideout just behind the edge of the dense forest on the opposite side of the river. That way they have a good view of the meadow. I will sit in the meadow, half-hidden by the grass. And wait. It's just about five in the afternoon and the tide is ebbing. Based on experience, this is a perfect combination of time of day, tidal stage and the natural activity patterns of wolves. Falling tides that extend into the evening and especially the morning hours offer wolves the best opportunity to catch fish.

We wait. I stay in touch with Richard and Simon via radio. Six eyes see more than two.

When we open ourselves to a place, it comes to us and touches us through all our senses. The burbling in the river, the rustling in the branches, the constant chattering of the ravens and crows, the occasional cries of a bald eagle. The damp, soft earth of the meadow, the felicitous scent combination of salty air and lightly musty-earthy smell of the rainforest. Two sandhill cranes land elegantly in the clearing and entertain us for a while with their dancing flirtation and their penetrating, rusty cries. A pair of Canada geese waddles around the meadow in search of tasty tidbits, poking around in the soft ground with their beaks. If I were to make a move now, they would immediately fly off, honking loudly. If ravens are the radio of the forest, the geese are its guards. Quietly I observe their little tour.

And suddenly everything falls silent. The atmosphere reminds me of something – of the tension before something important happens, holding your breath before a big entrance, an end to waiting. Slowly I lift my binoculars to my eyes and once again begin to carefully scan the edge of the forest for any movement, any tiny change. Then my radio crackles: "Wolf, centre left," Richard hisses. I turn my binoculars in that direction just as the first animal steps into the clearing. Fascinated, I focus my gaze on the forest again as the next and then another wolf right behind it become visible. In the end, there are six adult wolves. The two parents are easy to recognize. They exude a calm self-confidence and are the leaders of the family. The head she-wolf turns her steps directly toward me. I have laid myself flat in the grass in the meantime. I don't want to force anything, botch anything, make any decisions. It is the wolves who have already decided to come to me. They determine the pace of their approach, how close – and how it will end. And for a certain reason I let everything unfold in perfect calmness. That reason is trust – trust in the situation and its main characters. Trust that the wolves will behave cautiously and thoughtfully, curious to neutral. Because that is how I have experienced them in my observations over the past years.

The parents circle me. I talk to them in a quiet, soothing, even voice to reassure them, but especially myself. And yet – there's no better way to describe it in words – there is something in the air that gives me a deep sense that everything is fine. A kind of instinctive trust that has been awakened through my work and my encounters with wolves. A buried memory and deep human longing for a paradise in which we once lived in harmony – with all animals as well. Whether this condition ever existed or will has no bearing on my certainty. This sense strips time of its significance; during the following experience, it ceases to exist. Later I have to ask Richard how long I sat there in the meadow with the wolves.

The lead female has come closer. I perceive her with all my senses – hear her breath, feel her gentle steps, smell her fur, see her face. Then she gives my leg a light nudge. Gently touched by the wild wolf.

There are no words to describe the state I'm in. I only know that I've never felt so alive, so human, and at the same time so much a part of nature. So big and so small. So me.

The wolf provokes me. She stands her ground in front of me and through territorial scratching with her front paws shows me who is in charge here. Her partner makes a more practical gesture and lifts his leg. Soon, though, both of the parent wolves have judged me not to be a threat, and that gives their offspring of the previous year a green light. Now the younger ones also come very close to get a better impression of the unfamiliar thing in the meadow. But none of them dares to come as close to me as the she-wolf did. Before long, the young wolves go back to their business and play contentedly in the open space. The mother, however, lies down near me, unperturbed, her partner a few metres diagonally behind her. Although she lies curled up in the grass, I notice how her ears twitch a little at even the slightest sound. Wolves are masters of efficiency. Finally she rises, slowly strolls over to her partner and insistently animates him to play with her. I sit upright. Alone among the wolves. The images before my eyes are unbelievable, but over the years they will slowly start to fade. My feelings, on the other hand, remain as strong and as real as they were in those moments when I actually spent an afternoon with a pack of wild wolves on an isolated island off the Pacific Coast.

To the present day I've never experienced anything comparable; nothing else is such an inexhaustible source of strength, optimism and my great trust that challenges will have a good outcome. Nothing has touched me so lastingly.

WOLF SPIRIT 10
NOVEMBER 2005

Over and over again I watch the recording of the wolf encounter in the coastal rainforest on the laptop next to my hospital bed. And feel everything again, and I feel so alive. Lone Wolf of the wolf clan of the Heiltsuk First Nations once said:

A wolf won't show itself unless it is trying to tell you something.

Every person has their spirit animal, their protective creature that they can call on at any time and ask for help. No, my spirit animal is not the wolf, but it is the animal that remains healthy through the presence of wolves and in return nourishes the wolf.

Get healthy again – this goal doesn't work for me. "Being healthy" is a condition so far removed from my current state of being that I can't even imagine what that is anymore. The term is too abstract, doesn't say anything to me. I need concrete goals and reasons why I absolutely must survive this disease.

Pauline, a good friend and wise woman of the Heiltsuk community, sends me a letter:

> *Gudrun, your work yet to be done is paramount for the healing of the Earth.*

For I, like every other human being, have been given a purpose, along with the trust that I will recognize it and fulfill it. This sentence makes me conscious of that purpose again, and this very sentence will become the most important one of all during the years of becoming healthy again. I still have something to do, something important and healing for this planet. That's why I absolutely cannot go yet, and that's why I can also trust in the endless healing power of the universe, the Great Spirit that unites everything.

My friend Carol visited me on the day after my operation. Although I can't remember it, she has been near me ever since with her handmade card. In the middle of a background with simple silhouettes of flowers stands one word:

> Loved.

That card stands right next to the one from my friend Astrid:

> *Always know in your heart that you are far bigger than anything that can happen to you. – Dan Zadra*

These lines become my mantras; they strengthen my inner vitality and convince me that something great is yet to come beyond the illness. At the beginning they are just my strategies for survival, but over the years they are increasingly internalized, give me purpose and hope for my healing, and later help me again and again to find my future direction.

Of course, there are countless setbacks during this period of returning to health, and there is frustration and doubt. Pauline has good advice again:

> *Gudrun, when the fear comes, look it in the face and tell it to get lost, you won't be possessed or dragged down by it anymore. That takes away its power.*

And often the fear does sneak in, most often in tandem with its sisters, darkness and loneliness. Then I have to consciously call on my "inner wolf" to have enough strength to brace myself against them. My body is no help at all during these many months – actually during almost three entire years. Its constant pain and its weakness interfere with my will, numb it for long stretches. For months, I lie on the couch in Phil's living room and stare out the window, as if through a veil, at the snow-covered mountains in the distance. I see "Sleeping Beauty," a mountain silhouette that is clearly the image of a reclined woman with long hair drawn against the sky. And I think to myself, no, I definitely don't want to lie around that long.

Everything is Possible

NIPIKA

"Welcome to Nipika." The big sign carved out of a piece of raw wood stands in the middle of nowhere. After navigating 14.5 kilometres of bumpy Settlers Road, the sign relieves drivers of their fear of being run over by one of the trucks thundering in the opposite direction, heavily laden with tree trunks or huge blocks of magnesite. And their concerns for their own vehicles, jolting from one pothole to the next through a cloud of dust that recalls a desert sandstorm. But then it appears, the Nipika sign. And everything is fine. No, not just fine, it's wonderful! Down a short turnoff from Settlers Road the dense conifer forest opens up and a large meadow comes into view; scattered around it are seven wood cabins and a larger wooden lodge. The cabins have been built with great care in the style of the first settlers, using roughly hewn tree trunks and white mortar between them. Bright blue aluminum roofs, red window frames and main doors. Each cabin is slightly different, but inside they are all equally cozy with Swedish ovens, kitchens, bathrooms and furnishings in Western country style. Anyone who finds their way here once will return.

Most guests are escaping from the big city of Calgary to spend a long weekend here. The place is perfect for that; you feel at home from the moment you arrive. No period of adjustment, hardly any rules, and lots of freedom. Nipika is Lyle's life's work, his dream, which he established with his wife Dianne and his son Steve with great determination, love and good taste. The wood for the cabins has never left the premises; it comes from the surrounding forest, for which Lyle has logging rights. Lyle mills the timber on a small sawmill in the meadow, and then he and Steve use it to build the spectacular cabins. Wherever the two of them happen to be working at the moment, you can hear their loud discussions from across the meadow: the two are like day and night. Around 30 years old, Steve is analytical, structured and incredibly fastidious; Lyle is the exact opposite.

When I returned Murphy to Lyle at Kootenay Crossing, he extended an invitation to come to Nipika. When I take him up on that for the first time, his family is sitting together in the middle of an unfinished cabin around a supper of packaged soup and canned beans. "Gudrun, we expect to have a good occupancy rate this summer, for the first time," Lyle says with delight as he slurps up the beans warmed up in the tin that he loves so much.

"Yeah, if we ever get the two cabins finished," Steve mutters.

"Of course we'll get them done," Lyle says, looking at his son reproachfully. For Lyle there is nothing, absolutely nothing, that can't be done. I have never met a more optimistic person. And he's very successful with that: he has already achieved a tremendous amount, but now he has arrived. He wants to make this place an El Dorado for nature lovers and sports enthusiasts, the top destination for cross-country skiers in the entire country, no, the world, the entire universe. Everything works out. The first UFO landings in the middle of the meadow, right next to the old wooden wagon, the landmark of Nipika, are expected any time now.

Temporarily, though, it will be perfectly ordinary people who want to be active and get away from the hectic pace of the city. Over the years, Lyle does indeed manage to design and create the most spectacular trails through his woods, along the Kootenay River, parallel to the Cross River and over bridges to waterfalls. In summer they become trails for hiking, running and mountain biking. In the meadow is a pond with a wood-heated sauna and a cedar hot tub. At the far end of the meadow stands the crowning glory, called simply "the Barn," again a result of a difference of opinion between father and son.

Father Lyle: "Steve, I bought the old stable down there in the valley. We'll bring it up here and turn it into something. It's over a hundred years old. I took a good look at it; the beams were all hand-hewn with an axe, and after all these years they still fit together perfectly."

"Daddy, you're crazy! That's a rundown heap of rotting wood. Forget it."

Today, with its elegant roof construction in the upper floor, the Barn is a showpiece, available to guests for celebrations, weddings, meetings or other events. On the first floor there is a modern catering kitchen, but also space for ski rentals and waxing, a room to warm up in and space to store horse equipment. Waylon, Gypsy and Eva stand behind the Barn in their forest paddock. On average three dogs and three cats complete the population of Nipika. Two years after my first visit to the meadow, I count as one of them. I am drawn to Kootenay Valley again and again, when helping hands are needed or when I just need a roof over my head in between research projects. When that happens, I either call the National Parks office and arrange the "deal" again – "You give me lodging and for that time I'll monitor wolves for you" – or I call Lyle and offer a similar barter – "You let me stay there, I'll help you with everything that comes up." The work at Nipika can be as simple as cleaning cabins – all the Wilsons help with that task because guests often move around on short notice when Lyle confuses an arrival or departure date again. But also feeding the horses, trail maintenance, helping with logging, and especially just being there. During the first years, the Wilsons still drove home into the valley late each afternoon, but with the increasing number of cabins and amount of machinery, they want someone on site to look after things.

I move into the little attic apartment above the workshop. In the first years, Nahanni and I are often the only residents of Nipika during the week. Then I enjoy the peace this place exudes and can really bask in its warm, homey atmosphere. The Kootenay wolves cross through Nipika more or less regularly, too. Topographically, the place is perfectly situated for that. It's like an island in the sea, because unlike the rest of the region surrounding it, no off-road vehicles are allowed here. And above all no hunting. Nipika shares a boundary with the southern border of the national park, where the long side valley of the Cross River flows into the Kootenay, which makes it an important travel corridor for all wild animals. Unfortunately, lots of hunters and trappers know this. When we're out skiing in the winter and come across traps, Lyle and I always urinate on them; the human scent is supposed to warn the animals. It's strictly forbidden to purposefully trigger traps.

The firmly packed cross-country trails are also easy and inviting paths for animals to travel. Time and again I discover fresh lynx, cougar and wolf tracks, and deer and elk are omnipresent. There probably isn't a single guest who doesn't see the bold elk and their calves on the meadow. Dianne quickly gave up trying to decorate the cabins with flowers; they always ended up as food for the elk. In the winter there's a daily meeting of the elk cows and their young at the horses' hay barn. The herd awaits breakfast, even though we try to make it uncomfortable for them. Rufus, the legendary Nipika dog with the orange-brown fur, is a master of antagonizing them while at the same time adroitly avoiding the sharp hooves of the adults, which are capable of killing any dog or wolf with a well-placed blow.

The many wildlife encounters give me the idea to install motion-activated cameras along the ski trails and summer paths. I would like to find out to what extent Nipika is truly "eco" and how the animals react to the increased presence of people. But my main goal is this: I want to find Hope, the former lead wolf of the Kootenay pack that I never see any more in the pictures taken by the wildlife cameras I've mounted in the park. Nipika sponsors the equipment, and in exchange I put together an evening lecture with the pictures and video clips. I want each guest to go home with something more than replenished energy: a little more awareness that the nature surrounding us, with its wacky surprises and often so funny faces, can impress us most deeply and lastingly when we really learn to see again. When people experience the natural world as entertaining and enriching, then taking pleasure in it and valuing it naturally follow, which in turn leads to actions taken to protect the natural world.

Lyle renovates the old cabin of the first settlers who cleared the forest and created what is now the Nipika meadow and turns it into a nature interpretation centre. At the same time, I take a course to become a professional nature guide in Banff and promptly have a new job. We haul all the interesting or special things we find in the forest, such as shed antlers or skulls, to the cabin, where they are displayed. The walls are lined with shelves full of relevant books, from stories about the settling of the area to field guides on regional plants and animals. And I convince Lyle that I absolutely have to have a good computer in order to present all of this professionally. The cabin is also the meeting point for my nature tours. In addition, we offer mountain treks to remote alpine lakes or colourful summer meadows that are dotted with fresh grizzly bear tracks. Way down in the Columbia River valley, the Columbia Wetlands are the second largest in North America. Only the Everglades in Florida cover a larger area. Here we roam the side channels with our guests, dragging the kayaks over beaver dams, picnicking on islands under the watchful eyes of bald eagles or searching the shores for traces of wildlife. But my favourite activity is still taking canoe trips down the Kootenay River. The river winds dynamically through the valley, which makes the canoeing experience fresh and varied. It is the lifeline of this landscape, and its banks serve many wild animals as trails. My eyes are constantly scanning the shores for animals, even though the river itself has its dangers, such as rapids or overhanging branches that demand my attention.

Nipika is the fulfillment of Lyle's dream. But without a group of investors, even he wouldn't have been able to succeed. Most of these people embody all that Nipika is: successful, human, familiar. Almost all of the investors live in Calgary and have some connection to the oil industry, like 99 per cent of the population of this booming big city on the edge of the prairie. Apart from the super high-tech mountain bikes on the roofs of their trucks and suvs, you don't notice their wealth. The core group are also good friends with each other, and many of them become my friends as well.

In November 2005, shortly after my brain tumour diagnosis, Mike, one of the investors, invites me to a café in Canmore. We sit facing each other at a small table in the quietest corner. Mike stirs his coffee thoughtfully. "Gudrun, a few years ago lots of us bought the right stocks at the right time. We've had a lot of good luck in our lifetime. We want to pass on our good fortune and do everything in our power to help you get healthy again."

"Thanks, Mike." That's all I can manage, because I'm tearing up. I know immediately what that means to me: Nipika – nothing is impossible. The Nipika spirit gives me support and encouragement. *Nipika* is the Ktunaxa First Nation word for "sacred place," for "Great Spirit," for everything that has healing power.

We hug each other and then Mike gets right back to business. "I'll look around for an apartment for you in Calgary, then you won't need to get a ride to radiation every day. Hopefully near the cancer centre and of course you should be able to have Nahanni with you." Mike makes phone calls and organizes. Later, he is not only at every discussion with doctors, asking intelligent questions, but he also does a lot of research into the disease and about the various therapies, and when I have to interrupt my chemotherapy, Mike finds a brain tumour specialist in New York who continues to help me.

Rob, another investor, invites my sister Gerhild to fly to Calgary using his frequent-flyer miles. A physiotherapist, my sister helps me find my new rhythm and plan for my life in the first few weeks. Investor Andy and his wife stand at my door with a bread machine, and when I'm doing better, investor Wendy, owner of the largest canoe and kayak outdoor adventure company in Canada, invites me to fulfill one of my life's dreams: a canoe trip on the Nahanni River in the Northwest Territories. This trip was one of the grand prizes in the big fundraising raffle that Nipika and friends from

Canmore organized for me. One of the investors won the bidding for the trip and immediately filled all the spots with family and friends. It truly becomes a dream, even if I am not fit enough for two weeks of paddling and camping in a lot of rain. But the special people in combination with the idyllic landscape carry me down the powerful river.

Nipika becomes one of the essential building blocks in my life. Especially during the time when many plans I had for my life fall apart. The builders of Nipika bend over with me to pick up the pieces and slowly put them together again. I owe my life to you and your attitude toward life.

WOLF SPIRIT 11
CHRISTMAS 2005

It's a quiet celebration with just a few friends and Gerhild in Phil's apartment. Not long ago my friends, spearheaded by Jenn, a sweet friend from Canmore, organized a big fundraising party at the Canmore Nordic Centre. The location is symbolic. This is where the 1988 Olympic cross-country competitions were held, with some brilliant victories. My friends promote the fundraising event with posters along the streets and in stores, as well as newspaper ads. Lots of people come, donate and auction things off. The success of it is staggering to me. It's not just that the generous donations and auctions raise a lot of money for my treatments and living expenses; beyond that, every single dollar donated also carries a healing, appreciative thought. The theme of the party is Retro Ski Bunny, and the costumes are crazy. I wonder in what basements and attics people found their classic ski jackets in neon colours and skin-tight ski pants from the 1980s. I get to relive all of it a few days after the fact, lying on my couch. EJ, a friend, has captured it all on videotape. I'm not allowed to be there myself – too many people. My immune system has shut down; the chemotherapy has destroyed my body's defence mechanisms. At the moment, it's vitally important that I not catch any of the viruses or other germs flying around out there.

Soon after this, my lab results sound the alarm again. My platelet count is dangerously low, which means my blood would not clot to close even the smallest of wounds. After some discussion, I decide to discontinue chemotherapy after five weeks, after 20 of the planned 32 sessions. I know my body won't make it through the entire regime. On the other hand, my team of doctors impresses on me that this will greatly reduce the effectiveness of the treatment. Again Mike is at my service: "We've got to find an alternative." He does some research, and he finds Ralph Moss, Ph.D., a specialist in brain tumours in New York. He organizes a phone conference with Dr. Moss that also includes me and Lyle.

"Gudrun," Dr. Ross says, "In your case, there's only one therapy I'd recommend, what's called Newcastle disease virus therapy, or NDV. I know a doctor in Germany who provides this treatment." I take this suggestion as a stroke of providence. Germany. That's almost like going home. The man could have been in Kuala Lumpur, but no, he lives in Germany, and even better, in Bavaria. Still on the phone, I nod, even though Dr. Moss can't see that.

"Thanks. I'll do that."

The therapy is expensive. Very expensive. Once again, the Nipika investors rally, and through Mike they assure me, "No matter how much the therapy costs, we'll cover the expenses. We've set up a fund for you. Joe is in charge of it."

Money never meant much to me, but now it's becoming a key factor, and I'm grateful that I'm able to accept this kind of help. I call the doctor in Germany. After a long, friendly conversation, he adds, "So we'll see you in two weeks; we'll organize a brass band to welcome you. And one more thing: coming home is always good for the healing process." I pack my things. Lyle takes on Nahanni. A warm goodbye from Mike. A difficult parting with Phil. Everything is taken care of. Everything is fine. I'm flying home. Mutti is waiting in Salzburg. A few days later, I'm sitting in a train to Markt Berolzheim, where Dr. Arno Thaller lives and works.

Dr. Thaller is tall and slim. He only wears white linen clothing, and everything around him is natural. His laughter is loud and fills the room, almost as if it were a song. Even at our first meeting, I feel I'm in the presence of the Einstein of medicine. I know that in spite of his usual medical training, he's not a typical doctor. There is more to this man. He thinks about things from every angle. He combines classical medicine with treatments that are not yet generally accepted, antibiotics with homeopathy, injections with acupuncture. I feel I'm at the right place. My illness demands that I cross boundaries. The beds for cancer treatment are on the second floor of the old rectory; on the ground floor, Dr. Thaller receives patients as a general practitioner. It smells like ozone. Many of Dr. Thaller's own photographs, with poems he's written himself, decorate the walls. There is always a bowl of fruit – organic, of course – and next to it a pitcher of water that contains some energized stones. His assistants Tanja and Christine, as well as Michi the physiotherapist, are highly competent and complement Dr. Thaller's mindset well. They've organized a small apartment in the village for me. I live with the Färbers, a couple which always rents their little apartment to Dr. Thaller's cancer patients. By now, patients come to him from all over the world. Nevertheless, I am one of very few who go through the weeks of treatments almost entirely alone. Once Gerhild comes to visit, my best friend Gabi comes another time, and Phil even accompanies me once.

The days are strenuous. The combination of fever therapy with local hyperthermia – an intense warming of the tissue where the tumour is located – and the injections of viruses are exhausting. The fever, which is intentionally generated every day through injections and reaches over 40°c, is especially hard on me. Just like a regular flu, it's often accompanied by an aching head or back or limbs. My body basically generates the fever itself via intense shaking. This is often very taxing and, because of the seizures that accompany it, can be very painful. What helps a lot is the caring support, as well as the knowledge that this process strengthens my body's own resilience at the same time that it weakens the tumour cells enough that I can overcome the cancer. This makes it easier for me to endure what I must. No non-specific chemicals that indiscriminately destroy all cells. Instead, only natural weapons are targeted to the areas where they're needed. This fits so well with my philosophy of life. The treatment is as individual as people are. And above all: what's the alternative?

Between the intense weeks of therapy, I recuperate at home. Mutti and I take short hikes in the mountains.

Still in Canada, a student of my Heiltsuk friend Pauline calls me; she's of the Stoney First Nation at the Morley reserve, which lies in the foothills between Canmore and Calgary. The Trans-Canada Highway cuts right through this people's land, and the reserve unfortunately has a bad reputation as a den of criminality. But she asks me, "Gudrun, where do you live?"

"In Canmore."

She says simply, "Good. The mountains are healing." This sentence resonates within me. And my previous connections to the mountains through my home and my great successes in mountain running become even more profound and meaningful.

Even during the three weeks between the treatment weeks in Markt Berolzheim, I still have to get viral injections every other day. Right at the beginning of treatment, an arterial port was inserted under my left collarbone. The viruses are injected through this port so they can be transported to the tumour cells in my brain via the shortest route possible. That's why the port is located in an artery. I have to continue getting viral injections during the weeks I'm at home and especially later, when I'm back in Canada. There is solid scientific reasoning for this therapy, but only very few doctors use it. Germany is the only country in which the freedom of therapeutic decisions is anchored in the constitution. Austrian law also permits individual approaches to healing. But in Canada, I was dependent on assistance from people who administered the viruses to me even though it was not permitted there. I was only able to continue the therapy because of those people. Their assistance helped me to survive.

By my third year into therapy, my body has had enough. It develops an increasingly intense aversion to the port, which becomes infected. I experience complications, high fever and seizures. Finally, after three and a half years, the port has to be removed during an emergency surgery. It has served its purpose. And thus my virotherapy ended for good shortly before Christmas in 2009.

My body has clearly said, *I don't need it anymore*. Of course, I can't simply be done with all of this from one day to the next, not physically and certainly not psychologically. I will continue to occasionally have issues with lapses of concentration, dizziness when the weather changes, or sudden loss of energy. The sword of Damocles called cancer still hovers above my head. Except I've already experienced a situation that people would call "extremely improbable," namely when I was touched by a wild wolf in a meadow near the mouth of a river in the coastal rainforest. Now, I want to prove that in my healing as well, the improbable has happened.

Not quite half a year before the virotherapy ends, I already have a new medicine: my little son, Conrad Kimii. He needs a healthy mommy.

Rain Man

SPRING 2009

He fell from the sky. Like drops of rain. The name Kimii is Cree. An acquaintance asked his friend, a Cree chief, for a fitting name for my baby. The chief dreamt of rain that ran over his face like tears. "*Kimiiwan*," the chief replies. *Rain man.*

Suddenly he's there, without a lot of commotion. It isn't until the end of the fifth month that he makes his presence felt. When I have my first ultrasound, my friend Diana and I are both astonished by this little creature that's already so fully developed. Once I am aware of it, the pregnancy I experience is very short. And so there is little time to adjust or make changes in my life. When I find out, a bolt of joy runs through me. I can hardly believe it. After all, following the heavy doses of chemo and radiation and during the ongoing virotherapy, my body barely functioned. I walk to the nearest café and order the biggest piece of cake they have. Then I call Mutti at home in Austria. "Mutti, you'd better sit down," I begin.

She immediately interrupts, "Gude, not again!"

"No, no, I'm pregnant!" Tears of joy. I buy a bouquet of flowers and some chocolate in a heart-shaped box – wonderfully kitschy. I lay the flowers and chocolate on the floor in the middle of the foyer and eagerly anticipate the moment when Ryan comes home and stumbles over them.

We've known each other for a year now. *Long enough*, I think, *at our age we have a good idea what we want.* I met him last winter in Nipika. I was his cross-country ski teacher. Lyle and I led a cross-country skiing course for local people. Lyle sent me out on the course alone with Ryan while he stayed behind with all the others. And so Nipika is even intertwined with my love life – at least for the moment.

Before that, everything comes to an end in the spring of 2007. Phil is at the end of his rope. He has given everything he had in him, while I couldn't give him enough in return. Phil starts to criticize everything I say and do. And then the day comes: "Gudrun, I can't go on anymore. Wherever I go, the first question is 'How's Gudrun?' No one ever asks how I am. I'm exhausted. I notice that all I do is nag and pick on you. I don't want to, it just happens. I just can't do this anymore. And you're not the woman I met and fell in love with anymore, either. I think it's best for both of us if we split up."

Even though Phil waited with this confession until I felt somewhat better, I was still very weak and needed all my energy for the simplest daily tasks. I had no energy left to devote to a good relationship. This breaks my heart. In the months before the illness, we had even talked about starting a family. Now the sickness has even managed to destroy our relationship, which had once been so strong.

A few days later, Lyle pulls up in his big truck and brings me, Nahanni and my belongings to his place in Nipika. He is there for me as soon as he hears about our breakup.

Many friends are disappointed by Phil's decision. But even today, I don't have a negative word to say about him. He was fully there for me when I needed him most. He lived for me, beyond his abilities. I cannot judge him.

Besides, I'm back in Nipika. I can work when I feel strong enough and rest when I'm having not-so-good days, or when the effects of the viral injections are too intense, causing fever or chills. Over the months, the number of good days slowly increases. And by the following winter, I'm even able to teach cross-country skiing lessons again. Soon Ryan is coming to Nipika regularly after his work in the valley. The first time he stays overnight, I suddenly have one of those feverish shaking episodes, and he just holds me in his arms throughout the night. Then, at the latest, he's fully qualified in my eyes. The following summer we take several camping trips together. Ryan is an excellent fly fisher, and I love to watch his elegant movements.

Everything seems to fit.

Then the door opens. I hear Ryan's steps and notice how my tension is mounting. How should I tell him? We never talked about this before. Will he be happy? Ryan comes in, and I look at him expectantly.

"What's up? What's the funny look for?"

"Ry, you're going to be a daddy."

In the same instant I sense that from this moment on, nothing will ever be the same. I've never seen a human being in such a state of shock. Ry is incapable of talking, thinking, acting. "Gudrun ... I'm not ready for that yet," is all he says. But with that, everything is said.

The past years have toughened me up too much for me to break down and cry and feel sorry for myself now. And my own joy is too great. Nonetheless, at this moment, that joy lies shattered into a thousand pieces on the ground. Right next to the roses and the chocolates. Ryan hasn't even noticed them.

We decide that I'll return to Austria for the birth. There, at least, I have Mutti for support. I have to decide quickly; soon I'll be so far along in the pregnancy that I won't be allowed to fly anymore. Okay, I'll stay in Austria for a year, max. I'm leaving too many friends and intense experiences behind in Canada – beautiful ones and painful ones – for me to want to leave the country forever. Just one year, no longer. It's long enough, however, that I have to take Nahanni along. Such a long separation wouldn't be fair. Transporting her becomes a stressful nightmare. Highly pregnant, I sit by myself in the passenger cabin and can't think of anything but the "only baby" I've had until now. Before she got into the transport crate, I gave her several drops of Bach Rescue Remedy. She was the embodiment of a panicked dog until she disappeared from my view. Now I need the remedy myself.

When we are reunited in Munich, it's a spectacle for all the passengers. If dogs were able to do back flips, Nahanni would have done hundreds of them. Now it's time to arrive and get settled in the world I come from, which has therefore shaped me, so people say. But then came the nine years in Canada, and they were like an eraser: they removed a lot. Then, new things were written over the erased passages. I found myself. Now I have two months to find my bearings in my old home. When the baby comes, everything will be new anyway, and I'll have to start all over again. By myself. Nahanni shows me the way; she's my only constant.

My offspring takes its time, but we could only roughly calculate the due date anyway. Based on the length of the baby's femur and things like that. Ryan flies over for the birth. We wait. It rains and rains. Then the time comes and the little rain child enters the world. A boy, Conrad Kimii.

Babies and toddlers are like a bottomless pit: you pour your time into them and it disappears somewhere into a black hole. One year turns into two years, and then it's been three years in Austria. Every year, a visit to my adopted country, Canada, except for one. In that year, on a hot summer day, Nahanni, who is so used to the wilderness, jumps into the brutally contained river in front of my house to cool off – and doesn't come out for a while. When she finally does manage to climb out, she has torn two ligaments and a meniscus. Cost for the vet: a plane ticket to Canada.

Conrad will soon turn three. Since I returned to Austria three years ago, reports of the natural return of the wolves to Central Europe have become more frequent. I take that as a sign, not a coincidence.

In the meantime, Conrad grows a lot faster than hardened prejudices and fears about wolves can be countered and corrected. Conrad grows faster than people's willingness to give the wolves returning home another chance. And Conrad is learning faster than many adults.

When it comes to the topic of wolves, it will again have to be the new generation that recognizes the validity, as well as the necessity, of animals such as wolves. This poor new generation that we are leaving with far too many problems and from whom we demand the tolerance and adaptability that we were never willing to demonstrate. A generation that we are depriving of more and more nature, which hardly gets to climb trees or experience what a wildly rushing river or walking barefoot in a forest feels like, which never learns the names of the flowers blooming all around.

A generation in danger of losing its sense of nature.

But our senses are what make us human. They are our connection to everything that is natural, our response to everything that happens in our environment. They are a masterpiece, perfected over hundreds of thousands of years.

They allow us to live intensely, they provide us with a quality of life that satisfies us, and they warn us of dangers and allow us to survive. They could disappear within a few generations if we deprive our children of the chance to use them.

In the meantime, this phenomenon is already so widespread that it has a name: nature deficit disorder. It's not only a condition that results from an increasing alienation from nature, it also describes the terrible toll that results for us humans. Direct contact with nature is extremely important for a child's healthy development: physical, emotional and mental. Nature is an effective therapy for depression, obesity and ADHD.

A nature-based education leads to drastically improved outcomes in school, and it helps develop critical abilities such as problem solving, critical thinking and decision making. Childhood experiences in nature also stimulate creativity.[7] I will never miss what I've never experienced. But what I have experienced in nature remains deeply ingrained in me, more than anything else, like a treasure chest I can open any time I need it.

If my own treasure chest were not so full of moments that have touched my life, my illness would easily have defeated me.

My treasure chest is full. I am rich. I want Conrad also to be able

7 See the Children and Nature Network, http://www.cnaturenet.org.

to say one day, "My mama helped me fill my treasure chest." That's the wealth I can pass on to him.

To climb on old trees, to marvel at standing deadwood, to jump into naturally flowing rivers, and to find lots of traces of living nature in the snow.

We have a lot to do.

The pack invests a great deal of time and energy introducing the pups to their environment. It is explored with all their senses. Everything is observed, sniffed, poked and gnawed on. Familiarity with surroundings, recognizing prey and dangers, even anticipating what will come next: this is the content of the treasure chest that adult wolves fill for their young over the course of a year or two.

This kind of educational regime is also in the human parent's best interest. They know that offspring that are well adapted to their environment increase their own chances of survival, as well as the continuation of their genome.

A female wolf can successfully raise her young in places populated by people who encounter others without judgment and with open minds and respect.

I wish for my little Rain Man that he'll have the chance to go fly-fishing with his daddy, to stand in a free-flowing river and with a wide-arching movement catch a fish that has never been caught by a human before.

Epilogue

A young wolf sets out and leaves her pack in order to change something in her life. She doesn't have the status in her pack to reproduce, to found her own family and lead the pack.

In order to reach this goal, she has to forge new trails. She has to take paths that she has never travelled before and that her pack hasn't shown her. She doesn't know where the animals that she hunts travel or where to find water, where she can take cover and where dangers lurk. But she sets out anyway. She may wander hundreds of kilometres until she finds her spot, a place that offers her all of that and ideally a partner with whom she can start a family.

Setting out means change, and change means life. When we can't change anymore, we lose our drive to actively and attentively make our way through life. Our spirits and our souls become rigid, and our bodies just carry our empty shells around. When you start to not *want* to change anymore, you are old, and when you *can't* change anymore, you are dead, even if you are still consuming or still believing what the media tells you. You are dead because you've written off your actual purpose, the one that is intended for you and you alone: your contribution to make our entire world a little better. No matter how small your contribution may be, if it moves us in the right direction, it is enough. The right direction – that's another way of saying what we all know deep in our hearts: to respect, love and preserve life in all its forms.

Danke – Thank You

We humans are social creatures. We need each other like the wolf needs its pack. There are many things I wouldn't have been able to do on my own in my life. To all of you who have helped me with so many different things, I thank you from the bottom of my heart.

First and foremost, Mutti, Edeltraud, who exemplifies a kind of strength that lets me believe that challenges can be mastered.

Without Mutti, "Leihopa" Albert and babysitter Anita, I also wouldn't have had the quiet hours necessary to fill these pages.

I thank the many people who took care of me during my illness, who carried me and believed in me. I don't even want to think about where I would be if it weren't for you. The "recovery team" the size of the universe with Phil, who gave his all, with the doctors, especially Dr. Parney, and nurses at the Foothills Hospital, who got my recovery off to an excellent start, then Dr. Jay Easaw and his team at the Tom Baker Cancer Centre in Calgary; I felt I was in good hands with you. I especially thank Dr. Easaw for his tolerance for new forms of therapy. With the help of the happy nurses at the Canmore cancer department, Renate Weber at the Invermere and District Hospital, and later the care of my family physician of many years at home, I was able to continue and eventually conclude my recovery. I'd like to thank Dr. Thaller for his vision and steadfastness; he has given many so-called "hopeless cases" the gift of continued life with his qualities. All of these people risked going beyond the limits of "business as usual" for me.

This possibility only came about, however, through the spirit of Nipika, the place, the idea and the approach to life that's shaped by "my buddy" Lyle Wilson with his family and the Nipika investor group led by Mike Broadfoot, who literally shared their good fortune with me. I'm also grateful to my professor, Dr. Helmut Hartl, for his helpful herbaro creams.

Many people and associations gave me everything I needed at the time, with their words, thoughts, prayers and deeds, from fingernail painting to preparing meals to financial support. There is not enough space here to list all their names, but each one of you will always have a special place in my heart.

My proofreaders complete the circle of those whose influence in my life I am grateful for. Especially my wonderful editor, Heike Hermann, who guided me through my autobiography with a warm approach and just the right amount of free rein. And my personal proofreaders Ingrid Adlhardt and Andrea Aufmesser, who whispered valuable tips and suggestions for improvement to me, so that I could hold my head high as I sent these pages to the publisher.

Very special thanks to all my colleagues in wolf research. You have taught me so much, especially about deep friendship. I miss you greatly.

Thanks to Mother Earth, Brother Tree, Sister Wolf.

It has been a wonderful, even therapeutic, adventure.

—Altenmarkt, Austria

Further Reading

The Raincoast Conservation Foundation: www.raincoast.org

Visiting Nipika: www.nipika.com

Projects of the Miistakis Institute for the Rockies: www.rockies.ca

The therapies of Dr. Thaller: www.praxis-thaller.de

European Wilderness Society: http://wilderness-society.org